Applying Computers in Social Service & Mental Health Agencies:
A Guide to Selecting Equipment, Procedures and Strategies

Applying Computers in Social Service & Mental Health Agencies:
A Guide to Selecting Equipment, Procedures and Strategies

Simon Slavin, Editor

Volume 5, Numbers 3/4
Administration in Social Work

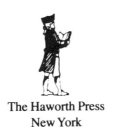

The Haworth Press
New York

The Haworth Press, 28 East 22 Street, New York, NY 10010

Library of Congress Cataloging in Publication Data
Main entry under title:

Applying computers in social service & mental health
    agencies.

    "Volume 5, nos. 3/4, fall/winter 1981, Administration
in social work."
    Includes bibliographies.
    1. Social service—Data processing—Addresses,
essays, lectures.   2. Mental health services—Data
processing—Addresses, essays, lectures.   I. Slavin,
Simon.   II. Administration in social work; v. 5, no. 3–4.
HV41.A66   001.65'024362   81-20102
ISBN 0-86656-102-1   AACR2

Applying Computers in
Social Service & Mental Health Agencies:
A Guide to Selecting Equipment,
Procedures and Strategies

Administration in Social Work
Volume 5, Numbers 3/4

> The computer is viewed as a tool, not only of management but of social work practice. The emergence of the "personal social services" as a distinct system, advances in computer technology, the development of computerized information systems, and the increasing use of computers in service professions and training make it necessary that social work administrators and practitioners become sensitive to the computer's capacity and potential. However, unless computers and the information they generate are meaningful and useful to service staff as well as management, their introduction will be resisted and their potential unrealized. Nor can computers be seen as solutions to more fundamental management, service, or social welfare problems.

> Information is a basic agency resource, and before an agency reorganizes the way it collects, processes, and reports information, strategies for improving its present information system should be carefully developed. The authors present a framework for strategy development by discussing the steps and activities in the information system improvement process, the associated organizational roles and structures,

the supporting tools and skills, the major options open to the agency, and the characteristics of successful strategies. An agency can use this information to tailor a unique set of strategies for developing its information system.

3. Management Information Systems and Human Service Resource Management 27

Glyn W. Hanbery, DBA, CPA
James E. Sorensen, PhD, CPA
A. Ronald Kucic, PhD, CPA

> *Creating effective, cost efficient human services programs is a major management task. The nature, extent, and quality of services are clearly linked to the financial capability and priorities of the funding sources. Thus, resource acquisition, allocation, and accountability must be viewed along with programmatic decisions within a context of intricate relationships. The Management Information System (MIS) may be seen as the cornerstone in any approach to overall resource management. With this view, the authors discuss planning and performance information, management of an information system, major management decision-making issues, and the context of a human services MIS.*

4. Feasibility as a Consideration in Small Computer Selection 43
Walter LaMendola, PhD

> *Feasibility is a critical step in the implementation of a formal information system, particularly one that will or does include computing machinery. Feasibility investigates and evaluates proposed systems, assesses costs and benefits of each alternative, and recommends system selection. Feasibility—technical, operational, and economic—is reviewed, and suggestions for moving through each feasibility step are presented. Attention is paid to the particular needs of human service agencies at each step, and examples are drawn from human service settings.*

5. Small Computers: The Directions of the Future in Mental Health 57
Alden C. Lorents, PhD

> *Small computers are going to have a significant impact on all organizations during the 1980's. The author describes some of the potentials of the small computer and its applications in mental health. He also cautions the reader regarding problems that are associated with acquiring these systems. The final section of the article provides information on significant studies that have been done and sources of information for those planning to acquire small systems.*

6. Managing for Success: Assessing the Balanced MIS Environment 69
Linda J. Bellerby, PhD
Lewis N. Goslin, PhD

> *The authors provide guidelines which permit mental health managers to determine the current stage of growth of the macro dimensions of their MIS environment. These macro dimensions are representative of the technical, managerial, and organizational behavior aspects of system development. A profile of MIS attributes for each macro dimension is presented. These attributes, derived from an empirical study of community mental health centers, distinguish among information systems at different stages of growth. The attributes allow managers to conduct a comparative assessment of the degree of balance in their MIS environment relative to experiences of other centers.*

PART III. APPLICATIONS AND CASE STUDIES

A computer based Decision Support System, judged to have successfully increased the equity of service distribution, is described. Aside from certain innovative technological features, the unique emphasis of the system is the creation of rules from below. Guidelines and standards move from the bottom up rather than from the top down. The authors discuss top down decision-making in In Home Supportive Services, design and operation of a decision support system, implementation and performance of a demonstration project, and the ingredients of a successful information system.

The authors describe the three-year experience of a mid-sized community mental health center in designing and installing an automated Staff/Management Information System (S/MIS). The purpose of the project, piloted at the Heart of Texas Region Mental Health Mental Retardation Center (HOTRMHMR) in Waco, Texas, was to examine the feasibility of a comprehensive data system operating at a local level which would create an effective audit trail for services and reimbursement and serve as a viable mechanism for the transmission of center data to a state system via computer tapes. Included in the discussion are agency philosophy, costs, management attitudes, the design and implementation process, and special features which evolved from the fully integrated system.

Austere funding, demands for monitoring and evaluation of service programs, and the need for information to inform decision-making have led human service agencies to establish computerized information systems. The service orientation of these agencies requires that information systems be developed and operated from a practice perspective, with consideration of the ethics and values underlying service provision. Case studies of information system development in two county agencies illustrate the application of this perspective.

Social service agencies are increasingly operating in a climate of greater demands for accountability. The author describes a working information system for a casework agency and describes the process by which it was designed. Using a system developed by the Jewish Federation-Council of Greater Los Angeles as the example, a model is presented for developing an Information System as well as a model for how such a system should operate. The development of the JF-C system is described from the first step of recognizing the need for information, through defining information requirements and setting up an administrative structure. Some considerations of systems design are included along with a description of reports and applications of the system to date. An evaluation of the cost-effectiveness of this system is provided.

HIPO diagrams are presented as an alternative to flowcharts and are shown to contribute to better problem solutions via the emphasis on top down and structured design processes. They are also shown to produce better documentation which will contribute to improved training and maintainability. The use of HIPO diagrams is illustrated with a presentation of the client tracking and services monitoring system in the HIPO diagram format. This example highlights the advantages of HIPO diagrams in producing readable and compact documentation of complex processes, and in implementing top down design and structured design concepts which provide module development (viz., Chief Programmer or team programming organizations) and module testings. The processes and concepts illustrated are appropriate for the design and documentation of a wide variety of human service entities.

A NOTE FOR THE FIELD

Applying Computers in Social Service & Mental Health Agencies:
A Guide to Selecting Equipment, Procedures and Strategies

EDITOR'S INTRODUCTION

The past few years have been witness to the rapid development of computer technology and its adaptation for a variety of purposes in large—and more recently—small organizations. It is reasonable to expect that in the near future the social agency that does not use a computer will be a rarity. Many have already been through the process of installing this new tool as an aid to administrative and clinical decision making. Many more are considering doing so. The essays in this volume are intended to provide a ready reference source for administrators who are thinking about the potential utility of establishing a computerized system in their organizations. They reflect the current state-of-the-art and lead one to anticipate continued and rapid technical development. They also suggest that the declining cost of instrumentation and programming might well make it financially feasible for the vast majority of social agencies to benefit both professionally and economically from installing an adaptable system.

As these essays indicate, we should avoid seduction by what to many appears to be an esoteric technicism. Professional training in sophisticated computer use has hardly begun to find a way into the schools which prepare social and human service managerial personnel. A few schools of social work have only recently begun to incorporate courses on the computer into their curricula. Practitioners already in the field tend to be neophytes in this area. This volume is addressed to those potential and practicing administrators who will perforce be making significant decisions concerning whether, who, and how to choose from the growing array of technical equipment. If the material in these chapters serve as an aid to wiser choices of hardware, software, and processes of engineering their use, it will have met its intentions.

Many of the following essays suggest the engaging of technically qualified consultants trained and experienced in adapting computers to organizational purposes. One is counselled here, however, always to bear in mind that technology must serve the purposes, values, and objectives of delivering services to consumers. Managers who are trained, knowledgeable, and experienced in the intricacies of service delivery play and indispensable role in planning, design, and implementation of technical resources. Furthermore, as experience in numerous instances indicate, all those in the organization whose

1

behavior is affected by changes in role performance need to find a place in the planning implementation process if any system is to have a chance of achieving its objectives. Computerization requires a sense of partnership, linking technical and substantive intelligence.

While the computer is a potent instrument, it can serve either negative or productive ends. If its use is devoted centrally to matters of cost containment in social programs and narrow concepts of accountability, and mainly directed to dealing with possible fraud and abuse, it can further punitive purposes. This is not to suggest that cost-benefit and accountability considerations are unimportant. Indeed, the computer can materially assist organizations to enhance efficiency *and* effectiveness and to develop accountability measures which grow out of the primary concern for service integrity and standards of performance. Where the primary orientation is to the quantity and quality of client service, the computer can be an aid, not an impediment, to the central objectives of service delivery.

Part I introduces the subject and suggests the importance of viewing the computer as a significant tool of both management and practice in the social and human services. Stress is laid on the importance of developing an appreciation of and sensitivity to the ways in which the computer can potentially enhance both administrative and clinical practice. Awareness of possible constraints on the utilization of this relatively new technical tool is also indicated.

Part II reviews patterns and strategies of information system development, issues in planning the adaptation of computers to social program agencies, and questions that require exploration in determining the feasibility of utilizing alternative system designs. The special requirements of human service agencies are suggested, as well as the assessing of costs and benefits of competing hardware and software claims. The unique contribution made by the advent of the small computer is detailed, and projections suggested for future developments in this rapidly growing and changing technology. Finally, the importance of understanding environmental factors that bear on the information system design, growth, and development over time is stressed.

Part III deals with special expectations and case studies of computer utilization. Some innovative departures intended to achieve special objectives are presented, as well as experiences in the use of computers for a variety of managerial and clinical purposes. Some significant examples are presented of developing systematic information systems which connect local and statewide data, as well as service information in a local social service agency.

It should be clear from the material in this volume that we are dealing with a potentially powerful and useful tool which can enhance competence in the service of organizational objectives. The immediate years ahead will undoubtedly produce new and experimental patterns in computer use in human service agencies. This journal is eager to provide a medium of idea and experience exchange on a continuing basis so that all managers can be kept abreast of significant developments in this field.

S.S.

1. COMPUTERS:
TOOL OF MANAGEMENT
AND SOCIAL WORK PRACTICE

George Hoshino, DSW

It is generally accepted that within the next five to ten years virtually all social agencies will use computers for much or most of their data processing and that staff at all levels will be directly or indirectly affected in one way or another by the increasing use of computers. The thesis of this paper is that it is the responsibility of administrators not only to recognize and exploit the capabilities of the modern computer for management purposes but to comprehend the impact of the computer on staff at all levels and to capitalize on the computer's potential to facilitate and enhance the work of all staff, including the front-line workers and supervisors. Thus, it is argued that the administrator must view the computer broadly, as not simply a tool of management but as a tool of social work practice as well.

Several developments have converged to make it essential that social workers be sensitive to the movement of computer technology into the operations of their agencies and appreciate the potential of the computer for their practice: the emergence of the "personal social services" as a distinct and increasingly important system of social welfare, one in which the social work profession plays a pivotal role; advances in computer technology that make computer applications feasible in virtually any agency; the development of management, or social services, information systems (MIS or SSIS), usually computerized, in social agencies; and the wide-spread use of computers in

Dr. Hoshino is Professor, School of Social Work, University of Minnesota, Minneapolis, MN 55455. Support in preparation of this paper was provided in part through a grant from the U.S. Office of Human Development Services (#18-P-00362/4-01).

5

service professions such as law, medicine, and education, including professional education.

The "personal social services" comprise a cluster of related facilitative, supportive, therapeutic, protective, and preventive services for families and children, the elderly, and such groups as the physically and mentally handicapped. Although services for these groups developed as specialized programs— and legislation, funding, and service delivery still remain largely specialized— there is growing consensus that they are parts of a larger system that is distinct from, but related to, the other traditional and well established systems of social welfare: income maintenance, health, education, housing, and employment.

The enactment in 1974 of Title XX of the Social Security Act, which provides for federal grants to the states for social services, symbolizes the recognition of the personal social services as a distinct component of social security for Americans, along with income maintenance and health. Significant features of Title XX are the requirement that services be directed at five specified goals, the emphasis on planning, and the specific references to needs assessment, accountability, and evaluation. At the same time, the personal social services are being consolidated into separate administrative organizations at the state and local levels. For example, in Minnesota the newly enacted Community Social Services Act consolidates into a single county-administered local outlet most of the personal social services and rolls into "block grant" federal and state funding for services, including Title XX, child welfare, mental health, aging, mental retardation, and alcoholism and drug dependency. The Community Social Services Act is similar to Title XX; it requires that each county and the state Department of Public Welfare develop comprehensive social services plans which must include a description of the method of assessing need, the services to be provided, unit costs, and the methods of evaluation. The Act, therefore, represents legislative recognition that a system of "personal social services" does, in fact, exist and creates the administrative structure and funding for such a system. Similar developments are taking place in other states, although exact forms and terms may differ. The significance for social work is that although many professional and occupational groups are involved in the personal social services, the social work profession plays the pivotal role in both administration and direct service.

The point is that what is emerging is a clearly discernible "personal social services system"—comprised of a body of rules, an administrative structure, financing, programs and services, facilities, and specialized personnel. The private sector is directly affected by this development because Title XX and other legislation authorizes public agencies to purchase services from private providers, creating a situation in which private agencies operate largely under public policy and with public funds, in effect, a quasi-public sector. It is possible, therefore, to think in terms of a personal social service delivery system as a total system and, in turn, of the system-wide information subsystem for generating and processing the data that make up the information needed by the system for such functions as management, planning, research, evaluation, accounting and reporting, and service provision.

The emphasis of Title XX, as well as other federal grant programs and state legislation such as the Minnesota Community Social Servies Act, on planning, accountability, and evaluation has led state and local agencies to collect data on a regular basis in order to meet federal and state reporting requirements and for their own planning, evaluation, and service purposes. Moreover, the data are individual-client, case, and worker specific and include observations on such variables as client characteristics, reasons for service, service provided, worker activity, and service outcomes. Even client perceptions of service can be routinely collected and entered into the information system.

The implications of the above are many. Although the conceptualization and definitions of the personal social services remain at a primitive level, a factor that compounds the difficulties of accountability and evaluation, the establishment of reporting systems and system-wide social service (or management) information systems has led to a degree of uniformity of definitions and standardization of units of measurement. The sheer volume of data and the reporting requirements have encouraged or made it necessary for most large agencies, and many smaller ones, to collect and report data in computer-readable form. The same volume and variety of data in computer-processable form has opened up new possibilities and challenges for the conversion of such data into usable information for management and services purposes. Given the volume and kinds of data stored in agency files in readily accessible form, "secondary analysis"—the analysis of existing data collected without the prior direct involvement or control of the investigator—becomes feasible (Hoshino & Lynch, 1981). Finally, the direct service worker and front-line supervisors become even more the key elements of the information system because it is they who supply most of the data on which the information system is based. The accuracy, validity, and reliability of the information produced are very largely a function of the accuracy and care with which the front-line staff enter the data into the system and that, in turn, is heavily influenced by the attitudes and perceptions of the staff about the information system, its component computers, and the ways in which the information is used.

Viewed as a tool of management and social work practice, the computer can be placed in a more reasonable and productive perspective: a product of modern technology whose potential and enormous capacity for processing data can be put to use in the interests of more efficient and effective management and better service. Currently, except for research, the computer has been used largely for relatively routine administrative tasks such as accounting and reporting. On the other hand, although still sparse, the social work literature on computers is growing rapidly and deals with a widening variety of applications including many directly involving client services and computer-assisted social work training (Abels, 1972; Boyd, Hylton, & Price, 1978; Jaffe, 1979; Rubin, 1976; Reid, 1975; LaMendola, 1979; Schoech & Arangio, 1979; Thomas, Walter & O'Flaherty, 1974; Flynn, 1977).

Agencies such as the St. Louis County, Minnesota, Department of Social Services, have developed systems in which workers directly enter data on clients through terminals and retrieve information for such purposes as preparing court reports and child placement. It is becoming almost routine for computers to produce the information needed by caseworkers and their immediate supervisors for caseload management, information and referral, and what workers previously maintained in their "tickler" files. Identification of community resources and probable eligibility for particular clients have been demonstrated to be technically feasible by using computers to match client characteristics with programs and eligibility requirements of social services (Adler, DuFeu, & Redpath, 1977). The use of "interactive" computers, by which clients directly interact with computers, is increasingly common, as for teaching CETA enrollees vocational and job search skills (Flynn & Patchner, 1981).

Information, whether computer processed or not, is an instrument of control, whether of program or, directly or indirectly, of staff. Because of the enormous data processing capacity of the computer and the use of computer processed data primarily for management purposes, front-line staff are burdened with increasing demands for more data but, ironically, they have benefited little from the management information systems and applications of computer technology. Indeed, when computer processed data are used by management for worker performance evaluation, the information constitutes a threat to front-line staff. Often they are put in defensive positions and react with hostility toward the information system, symbolized by the computer, and may even attempt to subvert or sabotage the system. These are not new problems, of course, but they have been exacerbated by the computer's capacity to process large quantities of data quickly and efficiently (Hoshino, 1973; Dickson & Simmons, 1970).

The administration of AFDC, in which reduction of error rates has become almost an obsession, is a case in point. It is well established that more errors are "administrative," that is, made by agency staff, than are attributable to recipients. It is relatively easy to design and operate a system in which errors can be spotted and attributed to particular workers and the information used to threaten or punish. It is more difficult to use the same information to prevent errors and to use the information system to assist the worker in doing so by identifying recipients. It is relatively easy to design and operate a system in which errors can be spotted and attributed to particular workers and the information used to threaten or punish. It is more difficult to use the same information to prevent errors and to use the information system to assist the worker in doing so by identifying recipients or areas of eligibility in which the probability of error is high, and to provide workers with timely information that alerts them to actions that need to be taken. In the latter instance, the data provided by the worker and processed by the computer become a tool of the worker's practice, as well as of constructive management.

In any discussion of computers in social welfare administration, the question of protecting confidential client information arises and merits serious consideration because of the kinds of clients served by social agencies, the problems with which clients seek help, the sensitive kinds of information necessarily divulged, the nature of the professional relationship which rests on an assumption of confidentiality, and professional ethics governing the professional-client relationship. Unless adequate safeguards are provided, there exists the danger of unauthorized access to or use of computer stored data. Again, the problem has always existed; it was not introduced by the use of computers although the data storage and processing capacity of the computer does add a new dimension. However, through the use of codes and access keys known only to authorized staff, computer stored data can be as well protected as traditionally stored information. Moreover, it should be kept in mind that if a person is determined to get certain information, he can usually get it through legal or nonlegal means.

The computer, however, cannot be seen as a panacea for more fundamental problems of management and service or a solution to social welfare problems. After discussing their project intended to increase the "take up" of various welfare benefits through a computer-based information system that provided individuals with personalized information about their entitlements to a wide range of benefits, Adler and DuFeu (1977) concluded that although the project was a technical success, it made little impact on take-up rates. The authors state:

> If there is one general conclusion to be drawn from our experience, it is that complex social problems do not have simple technical solutions, however rational these may appear to the technical experts. For such technical solutions to work they must be seen by those for whom they have been designed as a rational answer to their problems as they perceive them. . . . Thus, computerized information systems and multiple or combined assessment schemes are not in and of themselves solutions to the problem of low take-up any more than means-testing is a solution to the problem of poverty. This is not to argue that technical innovations can make no contributions to the solution of complex social problems. . . . However, they can only do so if they are introduced in a manner which is acceptable both to the implementing organization and to the user public (pp. 445–46).

In conclusion, one recalls the Luddites of early nineteenth century England who attacked and attempted to destroy the machines being introduced during the early years of the Industrial Revolution. To the Luddites, the machines themselves were the evil. The Industrial Revolution did bring massive upheavals to the social order but also led to the high standards of living of industrial societies and few would care to return to the scarcity and drudgery of pre-industrial society. Thus, the controversies over computers and resistance to their use can be seen as natural and inherent elements of the process through which a new technology is adapted to the purposes of social welfare, the social agency, and social work practice.

REFERENCES

Abels, P. Can computers do social work? *Social Work,* 1972, *17,* 5–11.

Adler, M., & DuFeu, D. Technical solutions to social problems: Some implications of a computer-based welfare benefits information system. *Journal of Social Policy,* 1977, *6,* 445–446.

Adler, M., DuFeu, D., & Redpath, A. *Welfare benefits project: Working papers 1975–1977.* Edinburgh: Department of Social Administration, University of Edinburgh, 1977.

Boyd, L. H., Hylton, J. H., & Price, S. V. Computers in social work practice: A review. *Social Work,* 1978, *23,* 168–171.

Dickson, G. W., & Simmons, J. K. The behavioral side of MIS: Some aspects of the people problem. *Business Horizons,* 1970, *13,* 59–71.

Flynn, M. L. Computer-based instruction in social policy: A one-year trial. *Journal of Education for Social Work,* 1977, *13,* 52–59.

Flynn, M. L., & Patchner, L. M. *Using an interactive computer system to strengthen retention and placement of CETA participants: The Champaign consortium demonstration.* PLATO inter-agency linkage project. University of Illinois at Urbana, March 1981. Mimeographed.

Hoshino, G. Social services: The problem of accountability. *Social Service Review,* 1973, *47,* 380–381.

Hoshino, G., & Lynch, M. Secondary analysis of existing data. In R. M. Grinnell, Jr. (Ed.), *Social work research and evaluation.* Itasca, IL: Peacock Publishers, 1981.

Jaffe, E. D. Computers in child placement planning. *Social Work,* 1979, *24,* 380–385.

LaMendola, W. A personal computer-based human service organization information system. *National Computer Conference Personal Computing Proceedings,* June 1979, 533–536.

Reid, W. J. Applications of computer technology. In N. A. Polansky (Ed.), *Social work research.* Chicago: University of Chicago Press, 1975.

Rubin E. The implementation of an effective computer system. *Social Casework,* 1976, *57,* 438–447.

Schoech, D., & Arangio, T. Computers in the human services. *Social Work,* 1979, *24,* 96–102.

Thomas, E. J., Walter, C. L., & O'Flaherty, K. Computer-assisted assessment and modification: Possibilities and illustrative data. *Social Service Review,* 1974, *48,* 170–183.

2. STRATEGIES FOR INFORMATION SYSTEM DEVELOPMENT

Dick J. Schoech, PhD
Lawrence L. Schkade, PhD
Raymond Sanchez Mayers, PhD

Computerization of agency information systems is proliferating rapidly as evidenced by numerous recent articles in the human service literature (Cohen, Noah, & Pauley, 1979; Elias et. al., 1979; Jaffe, 1979; Schoech, 1979). Television and magazine advertisements daily expound the capabilities and low cost of computer applications, such as information systems. Although information system and computer jargon is unfamiliar, the promises and potentials are enticing. Before launching into the uncertain waters of computer systems, however, some hard basic questions should be addressed. How does a human service agency move into a computerized information system environment, i.e., develop an overall approach or strategy? What processes and tasks are involved? How would it impact agency workload, staffing, and organizational structure? What tools and skills are needed? What options are open to the agency in developing this overall strategy? And finally, are there successful and unsuccessful ways to proceed?

In addressing these questions, this article presents generalized strategies that have been derived from years of experience in developing or improving information systems in a wide range of organizations. These strategies require consideration of the information system improvement process, the accompany-

Dr. Schoech and Dr. Mayers are Assistant Professors, Graduate School of Social Work, University of Texas at Arlington, PO Box 19129, Arlington, TX 76019. Dr. Schkade is Professor and Chairman, Systems Analysis Department, College of Business Administration, University of Texas at Arlington, PO Box 19437, Arlington.

ing organizational roles and structure, and the required tools and skills. They also require consideration of the options available to the agency in improving its information system and an awareness of the characteristics of previous successful efforts. Agencies wanting to improve their information system can benefit greatly by applying this knowledge and developing an overall information system improvement strategy appropriate to the needs of their specific agency.

The Information System Improvement Process

Every agency presently has an information system, since data is collected, stored, managed, and used in reports and for decision making. However, many manual information systems are no longer adequate to meet the increasingly complex data demands which are being placed on agencies. Often the data needed to make decisions is not collected, or if collected, it is stored in such a way that useful retrieval is extremely difficult.

Before changes in an agency information system can occur, the agency must begin to view the information it collects as a primary resource to be managed as other basic agency resources such as personnel, money, and property. Planning for the agency's information needs is a process as important as preparing the budget or anticipating personnel needs. Similarly, data collection, storage, manipulation, and retrieval require staff time and effort. A cost-benefit anaylsis of the information resource is advised to insure the output from the data management effort is worth the expense incurred.

The goal of an agency information management effort should be progressively to improve the existing system using available technologies and skills until the system meets the decision making needs of the agency on a cost effective basis. Achieving this goal may or may not involve computerization. For example, Figure 1 illustrates a small inexpensive manual system with many of the features of a computerized system.

The process of improving an agency information system is a major strategy consideration requiring significant agency time and effort. Figure 2 presents a sequential flowchart of the process an agency must follow to improve its information system. The process is iterative. Each step builds on and amplifies activities of the previous step. For example, the first step, preparedness and feasibility, must be given repeated consideration throughout the process.

Appendix A presents the activities involved in each step of the information system improvement process flowcharted in Figure 2. Each step begins with the planning of the goals, objectives, tasks, schedules, checkpoints, responsibilities and completion criteria. Each step ends with the documentation of all activities compiled into a report that is the basis for deciding whether to proceed to the next step. Completing this process for a relatively small agency subsystem may take more than a year, and it is important not to rush the process

Figure 1. A manual data system for a small agency

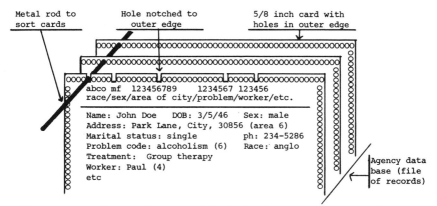

This simple manual system has some of the basic elements of an automated

system. Client data are written on a record (5X8 card) which is randomly

stored in the file of records which constitutes the agency data base. The

most frequently used data are recorded on the outside of the card by notching

the hole to the outer edge. Thus, each hole forms a key by which the data

base can be sorted using the metal rod. For example, all cards of anglo

clients would be notched to the outer edge in the "a" position above race;

all blacks in the "b" position, etc. Inserting the metal rod through the

anglo key of the data base and lifting would extract all races except anglos.

Additional sorts of the anglo cards could obtain all anglo males in a given

age group who reside in a particular area of the city, who have a specified

problem and who have been assigned to a given worker. Note that this system

is not a complete information system, for it only records, stores, sorts, and

retrieves data. A complete information system contains the people, equipment

and prodedures to collect data, perform more complex sorts and processing as

frequencies and descriptive statistics, and generate reports to meet user needs.

or take shortcuts. While going through the information system improvement process may appear to be a precise science, in actuality the movement through the process can be considered an art, and as some authors note, the state of the art in information system design is still primitive (Davis, 1974).

Each step in the information system improvement process requires careful consideration for effective development. Agencies may emphasize different

Figure 2. Flowchart of the process to improve an agency information system

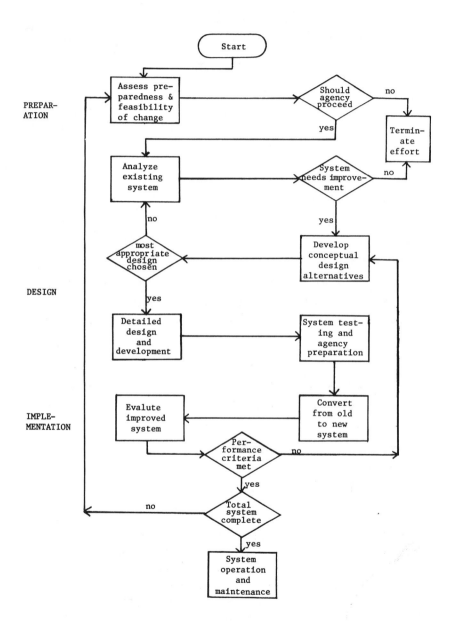

parts of the process depending on their specific situation. For example, an agency purchasing an information system from a vendor may skip some of the activities, especially in the design phase, because these activities have already been completed by the vendor. However, the agency should compile complete documentation on all activities no matter when, where, or by whom they were completed.

The major steps in the system improvement process are described as follows.

Step 1: Assess Preparedness and Feasibility

The first step is to determine if the agency has the motivation, capacity, and opportunity to proceed. This activity involves establishing communication channels to identify the extent of support and types of concerns, and to begin the crucial dialogue whereby the agency learns to develop realistic expectations of the processes involved and the results to be obtained.

The process of improving an information system is a major undertaking which takes money, time, effort, commitment, and trust. System change cannot be forced on the agency, since the success of an information system is dependent on accurate input of data by staff and the use of system output in decision making. The decision to proceed with the information system effort should be well thought out; however, hard facts rarely will justify the effort. Eventually the decision must be based on the belief that an improved system will be worth the time and effort expended, because it will allow the agency to better function, survive, and serve its clients.

Step 2: Analysis of the Existing System

Since data is a resource which flows through the whole organization, the study of its origin, movement through the agency, and use will involve analyzing all departmental forms and reports, data flows and procedures, as well as the decisions and goals which must be supported by data. The intent of this step is to gain an understanding of how the present system functions and to gather the information on which to base improvements. Since the existing system has evolved to meet the agency's needs, it should be a prime source of ideas for designing any new system.

Step 3: Conceptual Design

Step 3 involves the process of using the systems analysis of step 2 to develop several alternative system designs that can meet agency requirements using minimum resources. The intent of this step is to build a data model that matches or mirrors the functioning of the organization. Hardware and software options are investigated in terms of agency and design requirements, and the advantages and disadvantages of all possibilities are explored.

Step 4: Detailed Design and Development

The intent of step 4 is to translate the chosen design into a working system of data, people, procedures, logic, forms, data processing and manipulation, and equipment. Designing the data base is a technical process that involves coding and storing information to reduce inefficient and redundant data collection and processing while having maximum access and manipulation capabilities. If a computer is to be involved, the data base should be developed by someone who is knowledgeable of computer equipment. However, the usual tendency is for agencies to become over-involved in the technical aspects of the design and fail to develop other broader, integrative elements of the improved system, especially people and procedures.

Step 5: System Testing and Agency Preparation

System testing, or determining if the system performs as designed, is extremely important, because once introduced in the agency, errors are a frustrating waste of staff time and effort and threaten system credibility. The system should be tested with infrequently used data as well as routine high volume data. System testing is especially important for complex systems where many subsystems are integrated and perform core operations for the agency.

While open communication should prepare the agency for the system, certain groups such as operators, users, and others affected by the system must be made ready to accept the system once it is implemented. As with system testing, spending the necessary time and money for educating and training agency staff pays off with more trouble-free conversion and less resistance to change.

Step 6: Conversion

Conversion, step 6, is the process of moving from the old system to the new system. Since information is basic to all organizational functions, conversion means not only installing a new system, but integrating that system into the total agency structure and procedures.

Step 7: Evaluation

Evaluation involves creating a feedback loop in the information system improvement process, so system performance can be compared with design criteria and expectations. System success can be measured in several ways as the activities under step 7 in Appendix A indicate. Although evaluation is one of the last steps, it must be a consideration from the very beginning of the improvement process. Ongoing feedback is especially important in the operation and maintenance stage of the process, so the agency can continually insure that its information system meets the decision making needs of the agency on a cost-benefit basis.

Step 8: Operation, Maintenance and Modification

The intent of step 8 is to develop a smooth functioning system which continuously matches agency needs. Since no agency is static, system improvement is a never-ending process. The system must evolve and change with the agency, or it will soon become obsolete. The life of a system depends on the changes an agency experiences. Systems in highly volatile agencies may require major changes after 2–3 years, while those in very stable agencies may function well for 5–10 years with minimal change.

Accompanying Organizational Roles and Structure

In order to improve an agency information system, the agency must be willing to create the organizational structure and to assign the responsibilities necessary for completing the process of Appendix A. Several alternative structures for moving an agency towards information system improvement are shown in Figure 3. While the structure may vary depending on how the improvement process is approached, the roles of key participants in the structure are the same whatever the structure. Information system improvement is a process involving top management, the person or department in the organization designated responsible for data and information management (the information manager), technicians and specialists, and an agency steering committee composed of department representatives, usually department heads. If one of these roles or participants is omitted, the chances of obtaining satisfactory results decreases dramatically, especially in larger organizations (Appleton, 1979).

Agency management usually consists of the executive and associate director, the agency board, and advisory committees or representatives of the parent organization. The role of agency management is to provide overall direction and to insure the effort does not falter due to a lack of resources, e.g., funds. It must not only sanction the effort, but demonstrate its commitment to go through with the process. It appoints the steering committee, adjusts work loads to insure that the effort does not simply mean more work for those involved, and insures that lines of communication are specified and kept open. Agency management must remain in control of the total effort by balancing the conflicting needs of the others involved.

The steering committee represents the overall agency in the improvement process. Its involvement insures that the improved system meets the needs of

Figure 3.   Possible organizational structures to improve an agency
            information system

STRUCTURE 1

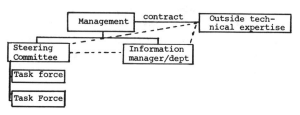

In structure 1, a balance of power exists between the steering committee
and the information manager. Disagreements are settled by top management.
Outside consultants provide technical expertise whenever needed.

STRUCTURE 2

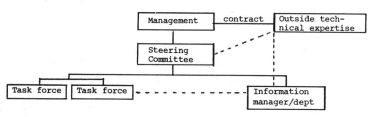

In structure 2, the information manager reports directly to the steering
committee rather than to top management. Outside consultants provide
the expertise needed.

STRUCTURE 3

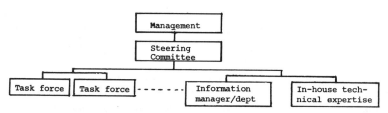

In structure 3, the steering committee makes major decisions and the
technical expertise is drawn from within the organization.

the overall agency. By definition, it performs an advisory role to top management, but it may be designated to have approval authority over certain reports or key decisions to keep top management from being bogged down in the more routine and detailed issues which must be addressed. The composition of the steering committee may vary depending on the nature of the subsystem; e.g., line workers would be involved in the process of developing a client information subsystem. The steering committee may appoint task forces to work on special problems or issues.

The information manager/department role may be a part-time job in a small agency or a full department in a larger organization. The information manager, often called a data administrator or a management information system (MIS) director, is responsible for managing and coordinating the information system improvement effort on a day to day basis. The information manager is ultimately responsible for the training that occurs and for documentation of the total effort. The information manager should be a top level generalist manager who understands all departments of the agency as well as the technical aspects of information systems development and should have the trust of and access to top management. The information manager daily manages the information system improvement process, while the steering committee sets the overall policy and guidelines and insures that the information manager's decisions are meeting the needs of their constituent departments. For communication and coordination purposes, the information manager should be a member of the steering committee.

Technicians/specialists supply the technical expertise needed in the information system improvement effort. The source of the technicians/specialists varies depending on the sophistication of the improvement effort and the expertise available within the agency. The technician/specialist may be an outside consultant, an information system vendor, or a in-house team.

Supporting Tools and Skills

The final consideration in developing strategies for improving an information system is the acquisition and application of a variety of needed tools and skills. These supporting tools and skills are described with references that provide additional information.

Planning and Scheduling

Planning and scheduling tools are necessary for guiding the project from start to finish in an orderly fashion. These techniques include the use of Gantt, milestone, and PERT charts (Carlisle, 1976). The design of control and feedback points in the process are necessary to insure that deviation from the desired course of action is detected and handled early (Burch, Strater, &

Grudnitski, 1979). Especially important is the ability to write clear, specific, and measurable objectives to guide and evaluate all processes involved.

Flowcharting

Flowcharting is the use of standardized symbols to graphically trace the flow of a series of activities (see Figure 2 for an example of a flowchart). Flowcharting graphically documents, simplifies, and illustrates the resources, logic, flows, decision points, and interactions of complex processes such as information system improvement. Standard flowchart symbols have been developed for the systems analysts and computer programmers (Burch, Strater, & Grudnitski, 1979).

Decision Tables

Decision tables or dynamic matrices which graphically illustrate complex steps of logic are used in information system analysis and design for study and communication purposes (Semprevivo, 1976). One common form of decision table is a decision tree where the trunk can be considered a decision problem and the branches are alternative solutions. Each major branch can have successive alternative or branching options (Davis, 1974).

Data Gathering Techniques

Since improving an information system may generate fears associated with technology, job displacement, job change, power changes, etc., data gathering can become a delicate process requiring skill and sensitivity. Good data gathering techniques, such as methods of observation, interviewing techniques, document analysis, questionnaire construction, and sampling methodologies are essential (Stone, 1978).

Group Problem Solving Methods

Information system development is a process involving groups, and effective group management is crucial to the effective system design and implementation. Techniques associated with such tools as brainstorming, nominal group process, delphi techniques, and conflict resolution are necessary throughout the process (Delbecq, Van de Ven, & Gustafson, 1975).

Training and Communication Skills

Communication and training skills help the changes associated with information system improvement occur smoothly. Miscommunication or lack of information can lead to rumors, fear, and resistance. Skills which help provide adequate information to all who will be affected by the system as well as skills in listening are especially important (Stewart, 1977).

Options in Information System Improvement

Numerous variations or options can be considered in developing strategies for the improvement of an information system. Some of the major options are outlined below, and references that provide more details are indicated.

Extent of Automation

Often the improvement of an information system is confused with the computerization of that system. The goal of an agency with regard to data is to have a system which meets the agency information needs in an efficient and effective manner. Computerization may or may not be a part of this goal. If a computer becomes a necessity, the agency must decide whether to purchase or lease a computer or buy computer time from a service bureau.

Which Subsystems to Develop

The agency must decide which data subsystems (i.e., service data, client data, financial data, or personnel data) are presently adequate and which need improvement. Some authors suggest that a system which is very important to agency functioning should be chosen for improvement first, so the benefits will be more obvious, while others recommend first improving a less crucial system in order to learn the process (Ein-Dor & Segev, 1978).

Source of Expertise

The agency must decide whether to develop the system in-house using present staff, to use a consultant to facilitate the system improvement process, to use a consulting firm to develop the improved system, or to buy a pre-packaged system. This decision is obviously based on agency funds, in-house expertise and the complexity of the system desired (Paton & D'huyvetter, 1980).

The Overall Design Approach Taken

The agency must decide if subsystems should be developed independently based on immediate requirements and combined into a total system when the need arises (bottom-up approach), or if a model of the total system should be designed first and each subsystem developed as an integral part of the total system (top-down approach). Each approach has its advocates. The top-down approach makes more sense theoretically, while the bottom-up approach seems to be closer to actual practice (Ein-Dor & Segev, 1978). A combination of both approaches is often a realistic compromise.

The Intended Users of the System

The agency must decide whether the system should address the needs of agency directors, mid-level managers, workers, or a combination of these. Different levels of the organization have different information needs (Gorry & Morton, 1971). Systems for data related to the more routine decisions of middle managers, e.g., financial data, are the easiest to design, while data supporting the complex decisions of caseworkers and agency directors requires the most sophisticated systems.

The Extent of Centralization and System Integration

Data can be collected, stored, processed, and retrieved at one central location or at numerous distributed locations. Both centralized and distributed subsystems may be independent or integrated to form one total agency system. The extent of integration varies with the number of different agency files and reporting requirements (Vickers, 1980). As files are integrated the complexity of the system increases, however the ability to obtain total agency data across programs also increases. The recommended approach is to design a system that reflects the extent of integration and centralization of the organization as a whole.

Converting from the Old to the New System

Four basic approaches can be used to convert from an old system to a new system, although a combination of approaches may also be used (Burch, Strater, & Grudnitski, 1979). The first approach is total or direct conversion, where the old system is discontinued and the new system implemented. Since this approach is abrupt, it is most suitable when the old system is significantly different from the new system and little carry over exists. The second approach, parallel conversion, involves operating the old and new system simultaneously until the new system meets predetermined performance standards. Parallel conversion allows a continuous comparison of the output of the new system with the old system. Running parallel systems is costly and it can be frustrating for staff to supply the data that the two systems require. In the third approach, modular conversion, the whole system is implemented in one section of the organization at a time, while in the fourth approach, phase-in or gradual conversion, the system is segmented and segments introduced into the total organization one at a time. Both approaches produce minimum disruption in the organization, but conversion can become a costly, frustrating, and a seemingly never ending process.

Characteristics of Successful Strategies

Factors that lead to success in improving an information system are a concern of practitioners and academicians alike. The literature contains mostly testimonials rather than controlled research. Identified factors have been cited repeatedly in the literature and can be used as guides for successful information system improvement (Bowers & Bowers, 1977; Ein-Dor & Segev, 1976; Schoech & Schkade, 1980).

As indicated in the discussion of the information system improvement process, one of the major characteristics of successful systems is adequate preparation and planning. Agency processes and procedures must be formalized and quantified and major changes made before developing an information system. Involvement is also key, in that top management must show commitment and involvement by controlling the overall effort and placing the information manager in a separate high level department. Users and others affected must be kept informed and involved throughout the process, since an effective information system is ultimately dependent on its users. Developing an information system should be a gradual process with one module implemented at a time and the total process well documented. Continuity of system developers must be assured, but this is especially difficult with the scarcity and mobility of well trained staff. Finally, all persons involved must be willing to handle the extra work and frustration required if the information system is to eventually result in improved decision making in the agency.

Conclusion

Developing successful strategies for improving an information system requires careful consideration of the information system improvement process and the accompanying organizational roles, structure, tools, and skills. Since an information system conceptualizes and operationalizes the core processes of an agency, the time and effort to develop effective improvement strategies must be taken, because a poorly designed and implemented information system is detrimental to agency performance and results in costly revisions.

This article presents information from which an overall improvement strategy can be developed. The approach presented is not prescriptive, rather it outlines alternatives within a development framework. The most appropriate strategies are those that combine general and theoretical concepts with the real world situation the agency faces.

REFERENCES

Appleton, D. A manufacturing systems cookbook, part 3. DATAMATION, 1979, *26*(9), 130–136.

Bellerby, L., Dreyer, L., & Koroloff, N. PREPARING FOR SYSTEM IMPROVEMENT; PLANNING INFORMATION SYSTEM IMPROVEMENT; MANAGING THE DESIGN OF SYSTEM IMPROVEMENT. Portland, Oregon: Portland State U. Regional Research Institute for Human Services, MIS Curriculum Development Project, 1979–1980.

Bowers, G. E., & Bowers, M. R. CULTIVATING CLIENT INFORMATION SYSTEMS. Human Services Monograph Series No. 5. Washington, DC: U.S. Department of Health and Human Services, Project Share, June 1977.

Burch, J. G., Strater, F. R., & Grudnitski, G. INFORMATION SYSTEMS: THEORY AND PRACTICE (2nd ed.) New York: John Wiley & Sons, 1979.

Carlisle, H. M. MANAGEMENT: CONCEPTS AND SITUATIONS. Chicago: Science Research Associates, Inc. 1976.

Cohen, S. H., Noah, J. C., & Pauley, A. New ways of looking at management information systems in human service delivery. EVALUATION AND PROGRAM PLANNING, 1979, *2*, 49–58.

Davis, G. B. MANAGEMENT INFORMATION SYSTEMS: CONCEPTUAL FOUNDATIONS, STRUCTURE AND DEVELOPMENT. New York: McGraw Hill, 1974.

Delbecq, A. L., Van de Ven, A. H., & Gustafson, D. H. GROUP TECHNIQUES FOR PROGRAM PLANNING: A GUIDE TO NOMINAL GROUP AND DELPHI PROCESSES. Glenview, IL: Scott, Foresman and Co., 1975.

Ein-Dor, P., & Segev, E. MANAGING MANAGEMENT INFORMATION SYSTEMS. Lexington, MA: Lexington Books, 1978.

Elias, M.J., Dalton, J. H. Cobb, C. W., Lavoie, L., & Zlotlow, S. F. The use of computerized management information in evaluation. ADMINISTRATION IN MENTAL HEALTH, 1979, *7*(2), 148–161.

Gorry, G. A., & Morton, M. S. A framework for management information systems. SLOAN MANAGEMENT REVIEW, 1971, *13*(1), 55–70.

Jaffe, E. D. Computers in child placement planning. SOCIAL WORK, 1979, *24*, 380–385.

Paton, J. A., & D'huyvetter, P. K. AUTOMATED MANAGEMENT INFORMATION SYSTEMS FOR MENTAL HEALTH AGENCIES: A PLANNING AND ACQUISITION GUIDE. Rockville, MD.: Department of Health and human services, National Institute of Mental Health, Series FN No. 1, DHHS Pub No. (ADM) 80-797 (1980).

Schoech, D. J. A microcomputer based human service information system. ADMINISTRATION IN SOCIAL WORK, 1979, *3*, 423–440.

Schoech, D. J., & Schkade, L. L. What human services can learn from business about computerization. PUBLIC WELFARE, 1980, *38*(3), 18–27.

Semprevivo, P. C. SYSTEMS ANALYSIS: DEFINITION, PROCESS, AND DESIGN. Chicago: Science Research Associates, Inc., 1976.

Stewart, J. BRIDGES NOT WALLS: A BOOK ABOUT INTERPERSONAL COMMUNICATION (2nd ed.). Reading MA: Addison-Wesley, 1977.

Stone, E. F. RESEARCH METHODS IN ORGANIZATIONAL RESEARCH. Santa Monica, CA: Goodyear Publishing Co., 1978.

Vickers, W. H. Source data processing. DATAMATION, 1980, *26*(4), 155–160.

Appendix A: Activities in the process of information system improvement*

STEP 1: ASSESS PREPAREDNESS AND FEASIBILITY

Communicate potential system improvement effort to all staff

Establish an agency steering committee .

Define agency ''preparedness and feasibility'' report purpose, objectives, timetables and responsibilities

Assess commitment of key individuals to proceed, e.g., board & ex. director

Assess motivation of total agency to proceed

Assess agency expectations of system improvements

Define tentative scope and goal of overall system improvement effort

Estimate cost & benefits, and time & effort for each step of the improvement process

Estimate improved system impacts (positive & negative) on agency & personnel

Relate improvements to agency's long range goals for information management

Write preparedness and feasibility report

Decide to proceed or terminate effort

STEP 2: ANALYSIS OF EXISTING SYSTEM (SYSTEMS ANALYSIS)

Define system analysis scope, objectives, data needed, data sources, collection methods, timetables, and responsibilities

Analyze current and future data input, processing, and output operations, & requirements of each subsystem of agency, e.g., forms, reports, & files

Identify major decisions made by the agency in normal operations and the data needed to support these decisions

Analyze present and future agency goals/objectives and the data needed to move the agency toward goal achievement

Describe logical routing or flow of agency data and data processing operations

Evaluate problems with the existing system

Analyze resources for change, i.e. money, time, expertise, etc.

Review systems in other similar agencies and request information from national or state associations

Develop policy and procedural changes necessary for system improvement

Prepare systems analysis report and preliminary design ideas

Decide to proceed or terminate effort

STEP 3: CONCEPTUAL DESIGN

Define scope, goals, objectives and checkpoints of subsystems to be improved

Develop alternative conceptual designs, i.e., possible flow and management of data, records, files and processing functions to match the data needs and sources

Apply agency requirements to possible designs, i.e., required and desired data frequency, volume, quality, privacy, turn around time, use and final disposition; and information system flexibility, reliability, processing and statistical capabilities, growth potential, system life expectancy, and tie in with existing systems

Apply agency resources to designs, e.g., money, time, expertise, existing hardware and software

Translate designs into equipment configurations and specifications

---

*For a series of workbooks designed to help an agency move through this process, see Bellerbey, Dreyer, & Koroloff, 1979–1980.

Detail the advantages, disadvantages and assumptions of alternative designs
Prepare conceptual design report
Make decision to proceed or terminate effort

STEP 4: DETAILED DESIGN AND DEVELOPMENT

Select equipment for chosen design
Design and develop the data base, i.e., processing functions and procedures, program logic, file definition and structure, keys and indexes, data error checks, storage and backup mechanisms
Set up controls and technical performance standards
Design input and output forms
Code and program system
Preparing operators, users and others to receive the system
Establish user priorities, run schedules, operating logs, etc.
Prepare programming manuals, procedure manuals and instruction manuals

STEP 5: SYSTEM TESTING AND AGENCY PREPARATION

Develop and approve system performance criteria and testing plan
Test input/output logic, programming, forms, and operational procedures and practices, and the use of outputs in agency decision making
Develop and approve a training and education plan
Educate and train system operators, data users, and others affected

STEP 6: CONVERSION

Develop and approve conversion plan
Incorporate information system into agency standard operating procedures, e.g., performance appraisals, new employee orientation
Reorganize agency staff and space if necessary
Conversion of equipment, data processing, and procedures
Insure all systems and controls are working

STEP 7: EVALUATION

Compare system performance with initial system objectives
Relate benefits and costs to initial estimates
Measure agency satisfaction with the system
Determine if system outputs are used in decision making
Examine if system improved agency performance, e.g., client services

STEP 8: OPERATION, MAINTENANCE AND MODIFICATION

Develop a statement of standard operating procedures
Prepare backup and emergency plans and procedures
Complete documentation, e.g., adding to, deleting from or modfying system
Outline a procedure for system maintenance
Begin step 1 if additional subsystems are to be improved

3. MANAGEMENT INFORMATION SYSTEMS AND HUMAN SERVICE RESOURCE MANAGEMENT

Glyn W. Hanbery, DBA, CPA
James E. Sorensen, PhD, CPA
A. Ronald Kucic, PhD, CPA

Managers of human service organizations have the task of acquiring and using resources to create effective human service services at a minimum cost. As part of this general management process, resource management focuses on the analyses, decisions, and actions related to:

—acquiring resources (or financing)
—allocating these resources (distribution)
—accounting for the utilization of these resources (evaluation).

The decision to add a new program or service, for example, requires financing. The financing decision, in turn, may influence (and may be influenced by) the mix or new staff to be acquired to provide the new services. The rate set for the service may influence utilization and third-party payment flows. The amount and kind of service actually received by the client is linked to the source of financing and to decisions on what staff will be expected to perform which services. The priority established by the state agency for a service, for example, may not coincide with the local priority, thus slowing or

Dr. Hanbery and Dr. Kucic are Associate Professors, and Dr. Sorensen is Professor, School of Accountancy, University of Denver, Denver, CO 80208. Portions of this article have been adapted from James E. Sorensen, Glyn W. Hanbery, & Ronald Kucic, *Accounting and budgeting systems for mental health organizations*. National Institute of Mental Health. Washington, DC: U.S. Government Printing Office, 1981.

hampering expansion of a service. Everything seems to be connected to everything else, and clarifying the full set of relationships necessary to making optimal decisions is difficult. In practice, usually some aspect of a given decision is examined individually and often one assumes the decision on hand has minimal effects on other decisions. Such practices can be dangerous—a series of separate decisions may work at cross purposes and produce bad results overall. Ill-tempered, simplistic one-by-one financial decisions can wreck effective programs, and financially unsound services and programs providing good client service can scuttle an entire center or agency. Concerns for both client services and financial management must be addressed at the same time if human service organizations expect to survive in the long run. A cornerstone in any approach to overall resource management is the Management Information System (MIS).

Planning and Performance Information

Management of a human service organization requires human service managers

—to make plans relating organizational goals and objectives based on the relative benefits and cost of alternative courses of action .
—to have control insuring efficient and effective action in pursuing the organization's objectives.

Plans and controls, however, require four generic types of information:

—planning information
    —what services the organization will render and to whom?
    —what resources the organization will use to provide these services? and
—performance information about
    —how effectively the organization is doing its job
    —how efficiently the organization is using its resources.

Role of the Management Information System

Developing the capacity to provide planning and performance information requires a management information system or more simply, an MIS.

Many human service organizations are just now becoming aware of the potential of information systems in planning and managing their activities. For many human service programs, planning has been almost nonexistent. The exigencies of launching programs, day-to-day program survival, and continuous funding crises have thwarted many efforts to engage in creative long-range planning. Consequently, most service programs have only perfunctory planning and development capacity; those that seriously attempt to plan find that events and programs seldom go as planned—something always goes wrong (although the consequences may be handled better as a result of their planning). Most frequently, planners and administrators fail because they lack the requisite information and corresponding information processing capability. Management information is the key to planning an activity, controlling its development, maintaining it on course, and measuring its impact. Management information systems have emerged as the principle tool for dealing with these crucial activities (Attkisson, 1978, p. 128).

The MIS must be dominated by what information is needed in decision making for the major questions faced by management.

The MIS must produce information that

—assesses the patterns of service delivery (e.g., who receives what types and amounts of services when and where?)

—defines how current resources are being acquired and being consumed (e.g., what are the major sources of revenue or what are the professional staff costs of the adult protective service?)

—provides monitoring aids for various human service providers and managers (e.g., were particular intakes inappropriate?)

—develops data for needed multiple reporting requirements (e.g., what reporting goes to funding agencies such as a state, Titles XIX or XX?)

—creates a data base for planning (e.g., are there changes in patterns of utilization?)

—assesses outcome of rendered services (e.g., what is the level of functioning of our clients and changes in their problems?).

Dimensions of Major Management Questions

Management requires select data on all clientele (usually less detailed) and on the resources acquired and devoted to providing various services (N.I.M.H., 1976). Managers at varying levels usually require report information focused around the five broad classes of information produced by the MIS. Usually, questions responding to external reporting requirements are completed from existing internally generated reports or by a search of an external source (e.g., census data).

Reports and Level of Decision-maker. Reports should be focused for the manager of a human service delivery organization. The type of variable and its measurement should vary depending on the *level* of the decision-maker. A report on each individual's percent of time spent in direct service may be

highly significant to an adult protective service supervisor but dims in significance for a legislator who is more likely to focus on cost per unit of service
purchased with state monies. Additional work is needed to flesh out the reports
appropriate for state and legislature concerns. Selecting and focusing the
measures for the level of decision-making represents one of the greatest
challenges. All too often detailed measures appropriate only for first level
supervisors are being reviewed by decision-makers charged with county or
state-wide concerns. The development of a well thought out hierarchy of
reports is needed to contain unnecessarily voluminous, duplicative, and ex-
pansive reporting activities. Table 1.1 attempts to illustrate potentially appropriate and relevant routine reports for the five major management questions
and for four varying levels of decision-makers.

Content of a Human Service MIS*

Interrelationships of MIS Content. The "management information system"
(MIS) is a relatively recent concept emerging in the last two decades. The MIS
generates data on all phases of operations including actual and budgetary
financial information and all types of statistical information. The role of the
management information system in *connecting the organization's structure to
the organization's process* is graphed in Figure 1.1. A natural product of this
formulation is a clear identification of *the vital connective relationships* among
the conceptual content of MIS, especially relationships among the conceptual
elements of statistics, accounting, cost-finding, budgeting, and outcome. The
elements of MIS are interdependent, mutually interactive, and are dynamic
over time in their role of connecting an organizational structure to its process.
The level of performance of any one content area is highly dependent on other
content areas in the MIS. If the accounting, budgeting, statistical, and outcome
data are adequately captured, cost-finding and rate-setting tasks or preparing
cost-outcome analyses are greatly simplified.

The planning and control reports produced by the MIS are the "eyes and
ears" of management in interpreting how the structure of the organization
relates to the actual activity (or processes) of a human service organization.
The reports are not equated with the process itself because of the abstractions
required to create understandable reports. The necessity for abstraction means
that some of the complexity of the actual process must be left out and this
deletion can (and does) lead to some distortion of actual program activity and
accomplishment. Reducing the complexities of a HSO to total cost of each
service and cost per unit of service compacts an enormous amount of detail

---

*Material in this section on the conceptual content of MIS is adapted from J. E. Sorensen and
D. W. Phipps, *Cost-finding and rate-setting for community mental health centers.* DHEW
publication No. ADM 76-291. Washington, DC: U.S. Government Printing Office, 1975.

TABLE 1.1

ILLUSTRATIVE REPORTS FOR VARYING MANAGEMENT ISSUES
AND VARYING LEVEL OF DECISION-MAKER

Major Management Issue	Level of Decision-Maker			
	Service Manager	Executive Director	State Department	Legislature
1. Patterns of Client Care & Services	.Time of day and day of week of admission	.Disposition of intakes by organizational service	.Clients discharged by major program	.Volume of services by service area
2. Source and Use of Resources	.Volume of service and patient load by individual staff (or staffing units) .Cost per unit of service	.Volume of service by type of service and organizational unit .Cost per unit of service	.Total % of staff time spent in direct and indirect service .Cost per unit of service	.Total % of staff time spent in direct and indirect service .Cost per unit of service
3. Monitoring Aids	.Admissions not meeting admissions justification profile .Listing of clients seen in 90 days	.% of admitted clients terminated without worker approval	.% of discharged ex-state mental hospital patients in community human service systems	.% of discharged ex-state mental hospital patients in community human service systems
4. Planning Data	.Volume of services for last three years .Seasonal variation in volume of services	.Volume of all services for last three years .Movement of clients from more to less intensive levels of service	.Level of poverty and historical utilization of services by Title XX clients	.Trends in use of various services
5. Client Outcomes	.Average changes in client functioning scores for specific services	.Average changes in client functioning for major target groups	.Ascertain existence and function of outcome evaluation system	.Ascertain existence and function of outcome evaluation system

about level of activity and resource consumption. Such computations, while simplified for ease of understanding, can be viewed only as crude representations of actual processes. Each of the major content areas makes its individual contribution to the reality simplification provided by the MIS.

Effects of Deficiencies. Deficiences in one or more of the conceptual elements of the MIS do not have isolated effects; for example, an *ill-defined organizational structure* coupled with an inadequate statistical content and weak accounting content will seriously impair the effort to do cost-finding. The consequences, however, do not stop at this point. If the Human Service Organization (HSO) manager cannot trace costs and delivered services to specific organizational units, the planning and control reports are deficient and, in all likelihood, so is the level of performance of the management team. Certain activities may be impossible; if, for example, budgeting is nonexistent, then forward (or planned) rate-setting based on *expected* activity and *expected* expense is nearly impossible.

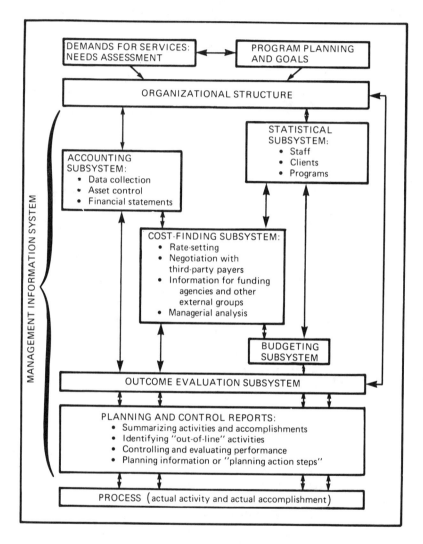

FIGURE 1.1

Source: J. E. Sorensen and D. W. Phipps, Cost-Finding and Rate-Setting
          for Community Mental Health Centers, National Institute of
          Mental Health, DHEW Publication No. ADM 76-291, Washington,
          D.C., U.S. Government Printing Office, 1975.

Data reporting systems are often designed more for external reporting purposes than for use by a human service organization's internal management group. Useful information can be furnished to both external and internal user groups. The questions asked by an HSO manager should be greater in number and detail than those asked by external sources. Most of the time external questions can be answered with summaries of existing internal reports. Certainly a manager of an HSO cannot ignore requests for information from those who are called on for financing the organization, but the manager should *not* design the information system to furnish only that information. Building a system for external groups solely can lead to a patchwork design with major gaps in information and reports as well as ineffective internal planning and controls.

Role of Key Variables

An effective management control system is intended to

—facilitate planning
—motivate managers
—measure performance.

The basic measure of profitability, a widely used measure in profit oriented organizations, is not appropriate for most human service organizations, but the concept of "breakeven' (viz., revenues equaling expenses) is a useful substitute measure for non-profit organizations. In addition to measuring "breakeven," the management control system highlights certain key variables that have a significant effect on breakeven. (These key variables are also known as key performance indicators, key result areas, key success factors, or just key factors.) The problem is figuring out what *not* to pay attention to so one can focus on what is really important. In most situations these key variables are few in number but are somewhere between three and ten.

Nature of Key Variables

Identifying key variables in a human service organization requires a thorough understanding of the programmatics and economics of human service services. These variables may be understood by discussion with persons who have a deep understanding and long experience with human service delivery systems. The important things experienced human service managers "keep an eye on" are likely to be the key variables. In general, key variables in mental health (after Anthony & Dearden, 1976, p. 139) are

—important to the success of the organization
—robust summaries of more complex relationships

—factors requiring prompt action when a significant change occurs
—sensitive to quick or volatile changes.

Sometimes key variables are measured indirectly by surrogate measures (e.g., client satisfaction by the number of complaints) but, in any event, they must be measured with relative ease.

Exception Variables. The current behavior of key variables always should be reported and scrutinized by management. Besides these key variables are a large number of other variables which may be reported if they behave in an exceptional manner—exception variables. Only when there is a significant deviation from plan is the exception variable reported. Under normal circumstances, the exception variable is not even examined or analyzed.

Identifying Key Variables

Each human service organization must determine its own key variables. Some, however, appear common to human service organizations generally. To make the concept of key variables more concrete for a HSO, for example, an incomplete list is offered below. The illustrative list is divided into three overlapping categories:

—Marketing
—Service Production and Logistics
—Asset Management

to make the analysis easier to follow.

Marketing. While many HSOs do not conceptualize or even believe they have a marketing function, it is there nonetheless. Usually some aspect of marketing is a key variable since significant changes in level of activity usually signal several other major changes. Illustrative major variables could include those presented in Table 1.2.

Service Production. In an ideal world, human services would flow smoothly, as calmly as a river normally flows between its banks. But, like a flash flood causing havoc and damage, unexpected events can damage the delivery system. Some variables deserving management attention and action to correct unsatisfactory situations include those in Table 1.3.

An Example:

One intriguing example of a systematic approach to capacity utilization and cost control is illustrated by Bexar (pronounced ''Bear'') County Mental Health and Mental Retardation Center in San Antonio, Texas. Over a three-year timetable the following steps were envisioned:

TABLE 1.2

ILLUSTRATIVE KEY VARIABLES IN MARKETING HUMAN SERVICES

Key Variable	Comment
1. Units of Service Rendered	1. Reveals shift in volumes or mix of services.
2. Revenues by Service/Source	2. Reveals changes in level of billings or other sources of revenue.
3. Scheduled Appointments	3. Assurance of future delivery of services is as important as current volumes and helps to assess if planned utilization of staff is on target.
4. Broken Appointments	4. While a variation on some of the foregoing variables, this variable identifies the level of lost opportunities to create units of service and may signal dissatisfaction with a service or therapist.
5. Repeat Clients	5. The return of clients who are expected to utilize intermittent or continuous mental health services indicates a dimension of marketing effectiveness; repeat utilization of those who are not expected indicates ineffectiveness.
6. New Clients	6. A surrogate measure of case finding effectiveness is the number or proportion of new clients added.
7. Uncompleted Treatment Plans	7. Early termination may signal staffing problems or inappropriate formulation of treatment plans.
8. Contribution Margin (Revenue less Variable Costs)	8. May signal changes in the mix of services or in proportion of services that cannot be rendered at regular rates; a shift in contribution may indicate change of mix of payors or eligibility of clients.

1. Determine a center-wide baseline of time accounted for in direct client or community service (initial estimates suggested about 25%).

2. Link planned increases in accounted for time to individual Management-by-Objectives commitments (initial increase might be in the range of 5% to 10% over prior year).

3. Provide timely monthly feedback on time accounted for in service and comparison with MBO commitment (accomplishments are expressed in totals

ILLUSTRATIVE KEY VARIABLES IN SERVICE PRODUCTION

Key Variable	Comment
1. Cost Controls e.g., • Cost per chargeable hour • Output per direct service professional staff • Overtime (or "compensatory" time off) • Cost per unduplicated client episode per year	1. Costs should be monitored all the time since the objective is often to only breakeven and a small change in costs can have a major impact on breakeven.
2. Capacity Utilization • % of time spent in client and community service • # of units of service per clinician	2. Unit costs and hence breakeven are influenced by volume because of the impact of fixed costs. Since staff time represents up to 80% (or more) of human service costs, chargeable time, which measures the percentage of total available professional hours chargeable to clients, is a key measure of resource utilization. If the available staff resources are not used today, they are lost forever.
3. Backlogs • # of days before receiving first service after admission	3. Expanding or contracting delays before clients receive services can be an indication of the need for a change in service delivery, e.g., reallocation of staff.
4. Quality	4. While most human service organizations take acceptable quality for granted, some measure of the output seems desirable. While difficult to measure, client outcome (e.g., global assessment) or problem reduction (e.g., Weed problem-oriented record) even if only on a sampling basis could provide highly useful insights about quality.
5. Yield • # of clients served • # of units of service provided and • # of units of service provided per FTE staff member (full time equivalent)	5. The number of clients served (duplicated) as well as the units of service produced by specific professional staff have an important effect on planned breakeven, and prompt action needs to be pursued when unexpected change occurs.
6. Fluctuating Costs	6. Any major cost which tends to fluctuate widely needs to be watched closely. In most human service organizations, labor cost is the largest but salaries or labor rates occur annually or semi-annually and can be taken into account without special signalling systems. Labor costs, per se, are not likely to be a key variable.

as well as percentage of target for month and year-to-date; current percentages are between 45% and 50%).

4. Estimate the cost per unit of the various services for each major organizational unit using cost-finding and rate-setting techniques described later. Unit costs include a "fair-share" of overhead. (The cost per hour of delivered service is one of the key computations since much of the mental health service is in an outpatient setting.)

5. On a clinician-by-clinician basis, compare the cost of the services rendered (viz., units of service times cost per unit) to a billing at a standard rate (before ability to pay adjustments or identification of third-party payor); report the "excess" or "deficiency" on monthly printouts of productivity. (The goal for long-run financial stability is for billings to be 200% of costs; by doubling the billings, accommodation of write-offs, provision of "free services," and funding program enrichment and expansion become possible.)

6. Identify caseload disposition on clinician's monthly report, with special emphasis on throughput and output of clients (the emphasis is focused on client productivity, and not client consumption of production.)

7. Identify client outcomes (e.g., non-financial but quantitative measure of change in client).

8. Link client outcomes to costs to perform cost-outcome analysis of various services and programs.

Asset Management. Breakeven is a function of revenues, staff, and assets employed in creating that breakeven. In human service organizations, and especially non-profit and non-governmental agencies, special attention needs to be focused on the behavior of current assets and liabilities. Table 1.4 offers four examples.

While the key variables in Tables 1.2 to 1.4 are only illustrative and must be tailored to the specific needs of a given human service organization, the concrete role of the key variable in signalling the need for prompt managerial action should now be firmly in mind.

Key Variables and Management

Planning and controlling human service operations requires measures of key variables. The interlace of management and key variables is conceptualized in Figure 1.2. By comparing budgeted with actual operations on

—client profiles
—services
—resources
—results
—special interest variables such as accessability, availability, etc.

TABLE 1.4

ILLUSTRATIVE KEY VARIABLES IN ASSET MANAGEMENT

Key Variable	Comment
• Cash (or near cash)	• Are cash balances kept to a minimum?
• Accounts Receivable	• How quickly are services billed? Collected?
• Inventories	• Are supplies and inventories ordered in cost effective lot sizes?
• Accounts Payable	• Are appropriate discounts taken when offered?

monitoring variances can be produced. Many measures are linkages of separate parts of the information system. For example, unit costs require a linkage of services (statistical) and resources (accounting) (see Figure 1.2). Cost per episode requires client services (statistical) and resource data (accounting and cost accounting). Other illustrative examples are depicted in Figure 1.2. External reporting is shown as a separate bar since, in most instances, the reports generally draw on summaries from internally generated reports.

Financial Plans and Controls

Plans. Successful organizations are characterized by good operating performance—efficient and effective acquisition and use of resources—and the genesis of this success is found in formal planning. HSO failures are frequently traceable to management's shirking financial planning, but in recent years the managements of HSOs have become increasingly aware of the merits of formal financial planning. The budget puts planning in the forefront of the HSO manager's mind and forces him/her to be a better administrator. A master budget integrates all of the functions of a HSO into an overall plan and highlights operating and financial problems early enough for effective corrective action. The master budget is the major point of departure for developing effective control of any organization.

Controls. The essence of controls is feedback. Comparison of actual performance with planned performance provides valuable attention-directing cues for the manager as well as up-to-date commentary on performance. Ideally, planning and control articulate in two interrelated loops as illustrated in Figure 1.3. Historically, the comparisons of budgeted-to-actual expenses usually show the current month and year to date expenditures matched against the

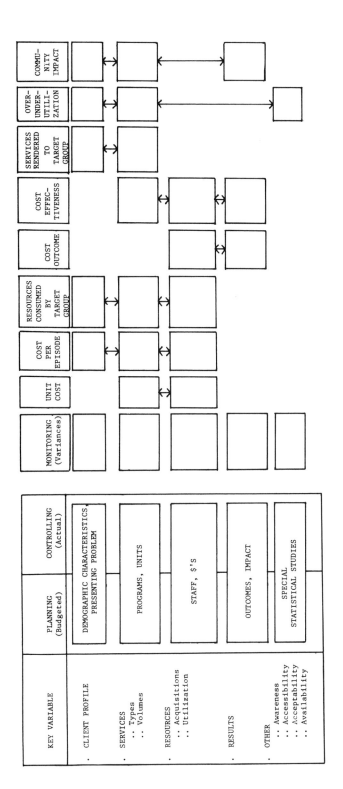

EXTERNAL REPORTING

FIGURE 1.2
CONCEPTUAL FUNCTIONS OF A HUMAN SERVICES MIS

Source: Glyn W. Hanbery and James E. Sorensen, "Using Information to Manage Human Service Programs", School of Accountancy, University of Denver, Unpublished manuscript (in progress).

PLANNING AND CONTROL

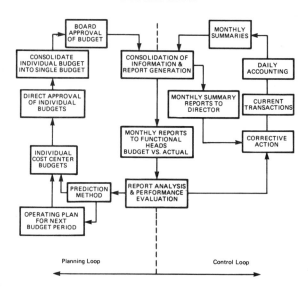

FIGURE 1.3

Source: T. S. Smith and J. E. Sorensen (eds.), Integrated Management
          Information Systems for Community Mental Health Centers,
          National Institute of Mental Health, DHEW Publication No.
          ADM 75-165, Washington, D.C., U.S. Government Printing Office,
          1974.

annual budget with a remaining budget balance identified. Typically, the
expenses are on a line-item basis. The master budget is static since it is tailored
to a single target volume of services; comparisons to the original plans can be
misleading if conditions (e.g., service volume) have changed. The need is for a
budget adjusted to the actual level of activity achieved—a *flexible* (or variable) *budget*. Flexible budgets are dynamic since they are automatically geared
to changes in volume. So the most appropriate comparisons can be made, the
budget is *reformulated* using the *actual* volumes of services achieved which
might be higher or lower than the original (static) master budget.

    If the HSO had an original plan, the top management might seek an
explanation of why the plan was not achieved. Knowing the differences
between the master plan and actual results may not provide a sufficient
explanation. Three major variances could provide a more penetrating explanation of organizational performance:

    —Variance from a *volume* of services target for a specific service (which is
labeled a ''volume'' variance)

    —Variance arising from changes in forecasted *prices* of goods and services
(which is labeled as ''price'' variance)

—Variance arising from changes in forecasted *use* of goods and services (which is labeled as "efficiency" or "use" variance).

External and Internal Pressures

Both external and internal pressures are shaping the joint consideration of human services and management information systems. While the allocaton of resources to quality service and good financial information may be delicate and volatile, the pressures for both continue to be expanding and unrelenting. An increasing number of external agencies request financial information; state and federal agencies, for example, are expanding reporting requirements for management information. Oftentimes purchase of service contracts are anchored in unit costing drawn from the management information system. When internal information systems are designed solely for external reporting requirements, valuable internal information may be overlooked or ignored. While the MIS must be responsive to external reporting requirements, the primary and foremost focus of the system should be internal since most external report demands can be satisfied with aggregations or reaggregations of data supplied by internally oriented reports.

REFERENCES

Anthony, R. N., & Dearden, J. *Management control systems text and cases.* 3rd edition. Homewood, IL: Richard P. Irwin, Inc., 1976.

Attkisson, C. C., *et al. Evaluation of human service programs.* New York: Academic Press, 1978.

National Institute of Mental Health. *The design of management information systems for mental health organizations: A primer.* By R. L. Chapman. Series C, No. 13, DHEW Publication No. (ADM) 76–333. Washington, DC: U.S. Government Printing Office, 1976.

4. FEASIBILITY AS A CONSIDERATION IN SMALL COMPUTER SELECTION

Walter LaMendola, PhD

The notion of feasibility is one that is critical to the implementation of a formal information system, particularly one that will or does include a computer. In computerese, feasibility refers to the process of *investigating* the present or proposed information system, *evaluating* alternative evolvements of that system, including the possible introduction of computing machinery, *assessing* the cost and benefits of alternative proposals, and *selecting* a system. Feasibility often includes the following steps: 1) producing a document called the feasibility study; 2) preparing specifications for vendors to use to submit bids; 3) obtaining bids; and 4) selecting a bid (Gilmour, 1978). In this article, the first step will be discussed.

Unfortunately feasibility is often poorly examined or even ignored. In part, this is due to the time and expense of feasibility assessment. In the human services, it is more often due to the onrush of events. An agency may suddenly find it has money to spend at the end of a budget period which must be obligated. Or, in those rapidly disappearing eureka days, a new government program appears with money priorities for information systems and a deadline of two weeks. These situations are handled well by the human services and very little money is turned away.

In an ideal world feasibility is an important phase in the life cycle of information system development. The cycle can be visualized as shown in Figure One. Notice that feasibility is part of a larger process. The life cycle

Dr. LaMendola is Associate Professor, Department of Social Work and Corrections, School of Allied Health and Social Professions, East Carolina University, Greenville, NC 27834.

process is continuous. The life cycle is iterative; in other words, the cycle does not usually proceed in a sequential manner from step to step. For example, the process may go backwards to a prior step as a result of new contingencies. The average time to go through the life cycle has been estimated at two to three years. The feasibility phase normally takes anywhere from three to six months. If computing machinery is to be purchased, add another three to six months to this phase.

Feasibility poses three separate types of questions: technical, operational, and economic. Technical feasibility is an assessment of whether or not the system under consideration is possible. Typical questions include: does a system already exist that can do this? Does the computing machinery exist? Are the computer programs already in existence? Does our organization have the resources? Operational feasibility defines the conditions which are critical to successful implementation of a system. Typical questions include: Will the system change the way we operate? Will the system change the way we deliver services? If the system is in place, will it be used? How will staff and managers adapt to it? Will the system meet resistance? Will the system be ignored? Economic feasibility examines the cost of development and the expected return in value. Typical questions include: Will the system save staff costs? Will the system save staff time? Will the system help reallocate resources? Will the system help develop resources? Can the system help the organization to do its job better? Will the system meet accountability needs?

This article will make a number of assumptions. First, it is assumed that the revolution of the life cycle under discussion will include automation for the first time. It is also assumed that 1) organizational management has given

STAGE	PHASE	PRODUCT
Definition	Information Analysis	Preliminary Statement of User Needs
	Feasibility Study	Proposed System evolvement
Structure	System Design	Specification of system hierarchy, parts, and relationships
	Program development	Programs planned, program needs identified
	Program Coding	Computer programs written and tested
Implementation	System Conversion	New system in place instead of or with old one
	System Operation	System use initiated
	System maintenance	Problems/changes resolved
	System Audit	Examination of performance

Figure One: Information system life cycle

complete and continuing support to system development, 2) a steering group has been established and will evaluate the information analysis, establish priorities, and approves system development so far, 3) a design review by (a) technical person(s) will evaluate the manner in which the system is being designed, and 4) an overall plan, hopefully developed with the participation of all staff levels, has been developed for the system effort. This means that there are written documents which, in a preliminary manner, define the system. These are important if not decisive assumptions. The success of computer machinery installation has been determined by top management participation and support, adequate planning and control, and effective action to deal with the human and social problems caused by the introduction of computing machinery.

The procedures recommended here assume a computer system for less than $20,000.00 is being considered. This price range is generally associated with the world of microcomputers today. However, the application, principles, and concepts must be honored in any case. The final assumption is that the person performing the assessment knows little or nothing about information system design, computers, or feasibility. The techniques used here are accordingly simplified.

Step One: Data Collection

Examine the existing information system by reviewing the materials of the information analysis. The purpose of the review is to identify the events that the proposed information system must represent in order to produce a benefit. Benefits in this case are expected reports. Use a format similar to the form presented as Figure Two. As events are identified, write them on one of the sheets and continue, ending up with one sheet per event. Once the review is complete, conduct interviews with staff around each event. The purpose of the interview is to identify what information needs to be provided, particularly that which is not being furnished. The event summary form acts as a face sheet to a collection of documents in use, proposed reports, and data collection needs for each event. These interviews and the completed event forms firm up the information analysis by ensuring a more complete description of the events which surround preparation and use of information. Data on expected costs is collected at this point. This is important, even though staff may say they have no idea of costs. An awareness that there is a relationship between cost and proposal is realistic and tends to help hold expectations to reasonable levels. The time span for information to be received back and the required level of accuracy are also items which can be estimated. All of this data will be important in the next phase of the information system develoment life cycle. When interviews are conducted, it should be recognized that many persons are not able to describe what information they need and use. the interviewer must

```
+------------------------------------------------------------------+
|                    EVENT SUMMARY FACE SHEET                       |
|  1.  Event description:                                           |
|                                                                  |
|                                                                  |
|                                                                  |
|                                                                  |
|                                                                  |
|  2.  Information needed back(time in days)_____Accuracy estimate___%  |
|                                                                  |
|  3.  What data needs to be collected about this event?           |
|                                                                  |
|  4.  What documents do you use to collect this data?  How often collected?  |
|                                                                  |
|  5.  What should the report(s) look like that you get back?       |
|                                                                  |
|  6.  How will you use this report?                                |
|                                                                  |
|  7.  Who will see and use this report?                            |
|                                                                  |
|  8.  ANTICIPATED COSTS                                            |
|         Personnel     _____                                  |
|         Equipment     _____                                  |
|         Supplies      _____                                  |
|         Other         _____                                  |
|                                 TOTAL $_____                 |
|                                                                  |
|                                                                  |
|                                                                  |
+------------------------------------------------------------------+
```

Figure Two: Event Summary Face Sheet

help them. In these cases, the interviewer will need to plan on more visits, mutual discussion, and agreement before completing the task.

Step Two: Data Refinement

Completion of the event forms leads to a comparison of these forms and their accompanying documentation with the preliminary statements of needs, sometimes called the information analysis product. If any discrepancies exist, they must be resolved before data refinement can proceed. In order to refine the data collection, each event must be reviewed and the following questions answered affirmatively: 1) Are all events which need to be represented by the information system described? 2) Are estimates for return of information and level of accuracy available? 3) Are there samples of all information to be put in the system? 4) Are there samples of all documents to be used for collecting information? 5) Are there samples of reports to be produced by the system? 6) Are there descriptions of how people intend to use the information they receive or issue?

The purpose of data refinement is to produce an overall verbal description of how information and documents will flow through the proposed system in the organization. The verbal description should be written in rather tight English. For example, a description of an organization's behavior planning system may begin as follows:

> The behavior planning cycle begins with the Initial Individual Program Planning meeting which must take place within 48 hours of admission. A plan is established at this meeting in order to meet the programming needs of the new resident. The meeting is set up by the Program Coordinator and attended by the core team, the new resident, relatives, county welfare worker, and other interdisciplinary team members selected by the Program Coordinator. The team determines immediate program needs and what baseline data should be collected. The date for the Annual Program Planning meeting is set and the interdisciplinary team is appointed for that meeting. Their level of involvement is determined for that meeting as either submission of an assessment or submission of a goal statement as well as their need to be in attendance. Copies of the Initial Individual Program Plan are sent to all named members of the interdisciplinary team. Copies are sent to the Program Director and the Behavior Modification Review Committee. The original is sent to Resident Records and filed in the Habilitative Programming section of the permanent record file. The second step in the cycle . . .

If the person conducting the feasibility assessment is familiar with flowcharting, it can be very useful to use the verbal description as a basis for a flowcharted data flow diagram (Davis, 1973). But accurate verbal descriptions are basic to any more sophisticated techniques and can suffice. In any complex system, it is preferable to write one verbal description of the information flow and one of the document flow for ease of examination and for clarity. In any case, a document flow must be written for each proposal that will move on to the next step. A number of alternative verbal descriptions can be written for proposed systems; each constitutes a separate information system proposal which can be winnowed out.

Before the proposal moves on to the next step, the document flow should be elaborated to include a data item dictionary. A data item dictionary records each data item on each document and defines its meaning, location, values, frequency of update, and collection. The dictionary may be kept on index cards and should contain the information on the form shown in Figure Three. The dictionary adds considerable information to help judge the feasibility of the system as well as contribute to the system design. The event summary forms and their accompanying documents, the verbal descriptions, and the data item dictionary are sufficient documentation to review the feasibility of a proposed system.

Data Item: _____

Short Definition: _____

_____

_____

Data Item Values:

If values are discrete   If values are continuous

Value   Meaning   Range of value Low_____
_____   _____   High_____
_____   _____   Length of value _____
_____   _____
_____   _____

(Continued on opposite side)

Documents item appears on
Frequency of collection
Frequency of update

Figure Three: Data Item Dictionary Card

Step Three: Technical Feasibility

Figure Four introduces the world of computers and computer programs. Computing machinery, sometimes called hardware, is shown at the top, with some examples, such as central processor and terminal. The rest of the chart depicts a variety of computer programs, sometimes called software. The system programs include an operating system, which is a program to direct and coordinate your system, and may also have a database manager as well as a program for sorting and merging. Utility programs are ones which facilitate use of the system. For example, the BASIC language is an easy to learn program which enables users to write their own programs. User applications are computer programs which have been written to execute specified tasks in the organization. A user application may be used for accepting data entry of client tests, analyzing the tests, and printing out the results. These programs, user applications, are the ones with the most meaning to the organization.

In the everyday life and needs of human service organizations, it is relatively safe to say that most proposed systems to meet needs are possible. Common sense can help you to determine whether or not that system is reasonable. There are five major areas to consider: 1) size of the data files containing collected data which is stored and maintained; 2) volume of processing; 3) single or multiple site requirements; 4) type of terminal and print quality; and 5) the availability of computer programs.

The size of the data files simply refers to the physical space planned to be occupied by the information you want to keep. This usually is calculated in bytes. For example, in a small computer, a byte is the equivalent of one character, such as an "A." One average page of text would contain 2000–3000 bytes. The bytes can be stored by recording them on magnetic surfaces, such as on tape or disks. Magnetic media have various limits, such as shown in Table One. Very simply, Table One depicts the cost relationship between storage media, storage space, speed, and cost. It is important to realize that similar relationships exist in every area to be considered. The costs shown are for one unit only. Any application will probably require at least two units, and a "hard" disk will require some type of unit for backup to prevent the accidental loss of information.

The volume of processing relates to the number of times you want to get on your machine in a given time period, the number of things you want to do at that time, and the method of doing it. If you expect to work the machine continuously, you may need to have the capability of having more than one person working at a time, particularly if different tasks need to be done simultaneously. Computers with a true capability to handle many people at one time presently cost more than the limit set in this article. The reality of microcomputers today is that you can expect to accomplish reliably only one task at a time on one machine. Microcomputer software is being introduced to provide

Computer System	
machinery	
central processor	memory
disk drives	terminal
printer	other machines
System Programs	
operating system	
monitor	database manager
sort/merge	dictionary
Utility Programs	
languages	disk status
transfer	dump
User Applications	
client testing	client tracking
staff time log	word processor
payroll	master file

Figure Four: Computers and Computer Programs

Magnetic storage type	Capacity (bytes)	Speed	Unit cost($)
5" Floppy disk	1-400,000	slow	500
8" Floppy disk	250,000- 1 Million	medium	2-4000
hard disk	10-73 Million	fast	4-7000

Table One: Storage media comparison

volume processing capabilities, but, as usual in the computer field, new developments should be approached cautiously.

A third issue is single or multiple site processing. Present microcomputers are distinctly oriented to one computer, one site. Their use of magnetic disks usually means that disks can be used at different sites on different machines. Also, there is great value to possessing more than one computer—which is possible and sometimes advisable at the low cost of micros—because machines break down. If one machine is not working, a second can be used until repairs are completed. On the other hand, multiple site processing utilizing only one computer is costly, more complex, more prone to breakdown, and should be undertaken only when absolutely required.

In addition to the computer and disk drives, the other machines you will probably require are a terminal and printer. The terminal provides a means for entering data into the computer. Terminals usually contain a keyboard for entry and a visual monitor for viewing entries and responses. The terminal can be very simple, but it can also be complex enough to be instructed to help the person using it. For example, pressing one key may be all that is required to load a program and execute a task; or, the terminal may be set up to catch errors and allow form editing prior to sending information to the computer. Terminals with added functions may cost much more than terminals with very simple functions. For example, costs for terminals may range from $600 to $4000 per unit.

Printers also vary widely in cost and quality. The print quality may be electrostatic; it may be dot-matrix, producing the typical looking computer print out; it may look as though it were typed by a professional secretary on a fine typewriter. Printers of medium speed (150–200 characters per second) which print out a complete set of dot formed characters will cost from $1500– $2500, whereas printers which produce camera-ready output will cost more. The fully formed character or camera-ready printers are also slow, typically operating at speeds of 55 characters per second or slower. In some cases, you may require one of each type of printer.

Decisions concerning machinery must be weighed not only by what you believe you require but what you can spend. A "minimum" microcomputer system that works off the shelf with computer, two eight-inch disk drives, a terminal, and a medium speed dot matrix printer can be purchased, without software, for $6000–$7000. However, added requirements can very quickly boost the price. For example, multiple site systems add costs for extra devices and for communication lines. In that case, telephone lines may be rented, modems or communication devices may be rented and installed. You must also have machinery at each site. This makes multiple site systems an expensive undertaking, and, of course, with more machinery and communication lines, more prone to breakdown.

Whatever machinery is purchased should be supported by the dealer through a ''service contract.'' Unfortunately service contracts do not always satisfy needs and have a kind of notoriety for their inadequacies. Nevertheless they are essential. All machinery breaks down, sometimes regularly. Only good service and, if possible, back-up systems, can protect against unacceptable levels of ''down'' time.

Computer programs are the final major area of consideration. Computer programs are sets of instructions which tell the computer what to do. The realm of computing machinery and programs have been generally discussed and are displayed in Figure Four. The area of concern here is the section labeled ''User Applications.'' These programs will probably total in cost more than the computing machinery. It is important to examine carefully the documents produced in the data refinement step, noting which programs might be needed and whether these are generally available.

The degree to which the programs you need are programs that everyone uses is one way of knowing that the programs are available and might work. For example, payroll, accounts receivable and payable, as well as general ledger programs are available. Some of them work well. Word processing and mailing label programs are available. Any programs considered must be clearly adaptable to your needs and meet your specifications or money and time must be committed to adapt or create the program.

In general Table Two outlines the relationship between cost, decision type, difficulty of organizational adaptation, and degree of information system ''formality.'' Decision type expresses the degree to which the rules for making decisions are either clear (structured) or largely intuitive (unstructured) (Simon, 1960; Gorry & Morton, 1971).

For example, payroll is structured; a decision to treat a client in a particular mode probably is not. Most human service organizatons have highly informal information systems with many unstructured decision making rules. It is this type of information system that is unlikely to have computer programs already available. These types of organizations fall into quadrant two: informal, unstructured, high cost, high difficulty. Some United Ways may be examples of quadrant four human services; however, there are few, if any, quadrant three human service organizations. Primarily this is due to the indeterminancy of their technology or, more simply put, due to the way they get things done. Small human services, which Hoshino calls garden variety social services,

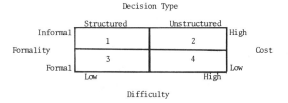

Table Two: Formality, Decision Type, Cost and Difficulty in
              Information System Development

probably fall into quadrant two. However, cost commitment is low because small systems can, in the long range, meet organizational requirements. The Table indicates why so few information system programs have been developed specifically for use in the human services. Unstructured decisions are most difficult to provide computer program support: informal information systems are difficult to model: in both cases, the cost is high. Available software is the key to a useful computer based information system, and the human services are only now developing that key. This is not to say that we are much behind the field. As *Datamation* pointed out in its issue on the eighties: "...software is something you can't see, taste, or understand—but it often smells!" Remember, most human service programs cannot be satisfied by presently available off-the-shelf software. This is pioneer country.

If each of the steps in technical feasibility has been approximated, a general picture of the resources required to get started should appear. If expectations and requirements can be made to fit likely resources, proceed!

Step Four: Operational Feasibility

Operational feasibility has been the primary obstacle to successful applications of automated systems in the human services. The question is whether or not organizational conditions will or can support successful system implementation. This can be understood by two dynamics: one, the problems pursuant to the introduction of innovation, such as documented by Rogers and others; and two, the occurrence of unintended or unanticipated consequences when the innovation is initiated. There are a number of strategies available here. Generally these concerns fall into five organizational areas: client, staff, supervisory, evaluative, and administrative. And, there are three related issues which deserve mention here because they will affect operational feasibility directly. These critical issues are confidentiality, advocacy, and service delivery.

Computer assisted information systems which utilize large centralized computing machinery have traditionally been opposed in the human services. One of the primary reasons has been the residence of client information outside the agency. With small computers, the information can now be maintained within the organization. Experience with small systems has shown that confidentiality can be protected at least as well as it was prior to the introduction of the computer, and, in most cases, with some degree of improvement. This is a major breakthrough in terms of the introduction of computer technology into the human services as this technology can be shown to support.

Another consideration of operational feasibility is whether or not it contributes to the agency's ability to advance client interests. Again, small computers adapted to organizational needs can support advocacy in fairly straightforward ways. For example, computer based files that can be used to produce reports telling workers when client services are due can contribute to client interests. Such reports will also provide paths of audit for supervisors.

Service delivery will also be affected. In each case, computer applications should be used to support important social structures. For example, if staff meet informally to compare notes to develop treatment planning, but were required to enter their notes in a solitary fashion on a terminal when the system got underway, service will be disrupted. On the other hand, clients may feel much more comfortable entering financial information to a terminal. In all cases, operational feasibility must consider these issues carefully and continuously.

Step Five: Economic Feasibility

Economic feasibility asks if the system will give a return in value that exceeds the cost of development: Will it save time? Will it help reallocate resources? Will it help develop resources? Can it help the agency do a better job? Will it meet accountability needs?

Most present applications in the human services have been developed to meet accountability needs in financial areas. This pattern of information system development is remarkably similar to the patterns of information system development in business. There have been a few major attempts, now becoming more numerous, to track persons being served by human service organizations and to audit services, primarily through counting procedures. The cost of these systems may run over one million dollars. There are also some attempts to build information systems from the workers point of view upwards. These are most promising for the long range. The gain in value from these systems is not only knowing whether or not the best service is being provided to a client but also the gain is 1) knowing what is being spent, where, and on whom, 2) who is being served and where they are in the service system, and, in the worker based systems, 3) what our experience has been with a person like this. When successful, these gains in information provide a foundation for managing a service or client; but these are intangible gains. In other words, knowing what is being spent does not necessarily lead to either better management, more available dollars, or a savings in dollars. Knowing past experiences with client, or where a client is in the service continuum may help the worker provide different, better, or required services if they are available, but, again, these are intangible gains. Intangible gains are more typical of automated information systems rather than tangible ones because the value of information cannot always be assessed in dollars. However, using the same examples, areas of tangible value can also be assessed.

For example, if the quarterly budget report takes one month to prepare and the information system prepares current reports weekly, there are obvious savings in staff costs. If workers check their caseload irregularly to see when clients need services and the information system prints current case status reports monthly, there are savings in staff time and in clerical time.

In order to perform a basic cost-benefit analysis, system specifications, as developed so far, could be sent to experts for estimates or to vendors for preliminary bids. Alternatively, the person performing the feasibility assessment could go out and shop around, gathering probable costs for systems which may meet needs. The information can allow for the construction of a cost table, as shown in the example in Table Three. The information shown includes costs for machinery, software, service and maintenance, training, and supplies. The costs are shown over a three year period, as if the expenses were to be borne as a part of a three year lease/purchase plan.

The second part of the cost-benefit analysis requires estimates of benefits in dollars. Benefit analyses in dollars squarely faces the problem of quantifying the intangible and qualitative benefits the organization expects to achieve. This has been and remains a major hurdle in the application of cost-benefit analyses in the human services. In other words, if one could measure client outcomes, how could they be expressed in dollars? Or, how are intangible benefits as well as qualitative benefits interpreted as dollar amounts? A pure, thorough cost-benefit analysis is probably not possible for the human service agency to perform. However, it is possible to establish a "minimum" benefit position for use in such an analysis. "Minimum" benefits are statements of the anticipated tangible benefits expressed in dollars. Usually, tangible benefits are expected in areas of office machinery and personnel. Personnel savings can be estimated in terms of full-time equivalencies (FTE). One FTE is equal to one-hundred percent of one staff position time for one fiscal year. For example, assume that the computing system will produce weekly budget reports using one-tenth of a budget clerk's time. The budget clerk estimates, or is observed to spend, sixty percent of time on weekly budget reports. The benefit in dollars can be expressed as follows: The present time commitment, .6 FTE, minus the anticipated time commitment, .1 FTE, equals a benefit of .5 FTE (budget clerk). The yearly position cost is multiplied by the FTE factor for each year of the project. In this case, if the first year cost for one full FTE budget clerk were $7874, the benefit would be $3937, or $7874 multiplied by .5. Since the salary would change each year of the project, the benefit would

ITEM	YEARLY COST			TOTAL
	1	2	3	
Apple 3 with hard disk	3600	3600	3600	10,800
Line Printer	816	816	816	2,448
Letter Printer	1245	1245	1245	3,735
Terminal	600	600	600	1,800
Operating System (CPM)	349			349
Softcard/Microsoft BASIC v.5	495			495
Magic Wand Word Processor	395			395
Peachtree Financial Package	2120			2,120
Installation	250			250
Service Contract	475	620	780	1,875
Training	500			500
Supplies	300	600	900	1,800
TOTAL	11145	7481	7941	26,567

Table Three: Cost Breakdown

increase in dollar amount. If the FTE savings changed over the project period, the figures would also be affected. It is also possible to anticipate increased costs as well as savings. A simplified ''minimum'' procedure, such as outlined here, was used to construct Table Four.

Tables Three and Four can be used to construct a simple but effective cost-benefit table, shown here as Table Five. In the Table, information concerning costs and benefits is drawn, each as a line. The shaded area of the table shows the time required for payback of the cost. A judgment can then be made as to the acceptability of the payback period.

In each case, evaluation of economic feasibility can proceed on the basis of the results of prior steps, particularly step two.

Summary

The advent of inexpensive computing machinery now allows for the expedient introduction of an intermediate technology into the human services. The garden variety human service agency is the perfect setting for the development of the application of such technology. Small computer systems now have the added advantage of a potential to meet past ethical, client, and service delivery obstacles to computer based system introduction. Feasibility is part of a larger information system development life cycle which investigates the present information system for the purpose of proposing the evolvement of that system. If human service organizations intend to take advantage of the unex-

BENEFIT	FTE	YEAR 1	YEAR 2	3	TOTAL
Personnel	.30	2362	3159	3350	8871
Client services	.25	1968	2625	2855	7448
Budget	.50	3937	5250	5520	14707
Quality Control	.20	1575	2100	2100	5775
Admissions	.50	3937	5220	5220	14377
TOTAL	1.75	13779	18354	19045	51178

Table Four: Benefit Breakdown

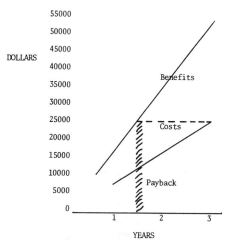

Table Five: Cost Benefit Comparison

pected opportunity to unite innovation and service, diligence and effort should be expended to determine the feasibility of their undertaking.

REFERENCES

Davis, E. *Computer data processing*. New York: McGraw-Hill, 1973.

Entering the eighties. *Datamation*, November 25, 1979.

Equity and efficiency project, first year report. Berkeley: School of Social Welfare, University of California, January 1980.

Gilmour, R. W. *Business systems handbook*. Englewood Cliffs, NJ: Prentice-Hall, 1979.

Gorry, G. A., & Morton, M. S. A framework for management information systems. *Sloan Management Review*, 1971, *13*, 55–70.

Rogers, E. M. *Communication of innovations*. New York: Free Press, 1971.

Simon, H. *The new science of management decision*. New York: Harper and Row, 1960.

5. SMALL COMPUTERS: THE DIRECTIONS OF THE FUTURE IN MENTAL HEALTH

Alden C. Lorents, PhD

Small computers are going to have a substantial impact on all organizations during the 1980's. The microprocessor on a chip, together with continued advances in memory development, is making it possible to have significant computing power available in various configurations from $250 to $25,000. These computers will be applied to various applications in mental health organizations over the next few years.

The typical configuration of the small computer consists of the following components:

1. The computer and memory.
2. A display device referred to as a CRT (Cathode Ray Tube).
3. A regular typewriter keyboard with a 10-key numeric pad and some function keys.
4. Some form of disk storage.
5. A printer.
6. Communications capability to connect to other computers via telephone.

The computer and memory are normally tiny components mounted on a board that is a part of the keyboard or the CRT. Memory comes in the form of RAM (Random Access Memory) or ROM (Read Only Memory). RAM is used to store general application programs, such as client accounting, while the

Dr. Lorents is Professor, College of Business Administration, Northern Arizona University, Flagstaff, AZ 86011.

57

program is being used. ROM is used to store system programs such as the operating system and the language being used. It is possible that ROM could also be used in the 1980's to store commonly used application programs in the mental health field.

The larger components of the computer system are the input and output units. The CRT, keyboard, computer, and two disk drives are all integrated into one unit in many of the systems today. The unit is not much larger than a regular computer terminal. The disk drives in these units normally use 5¼ inch diameter floppy disks or diskettes that hold from 100,000 characters to 500,000 characters per drive. Storage is normally referred to in K bytes or megabytes where K = 1000, mega = 1,000,000, and a byte is a storage position for a character.

Larger disks systems for the small computers use eight inch diameter diskettes that hold up to one million characters per diskette and eight inch hard disks that store up to 24 million characters per drive. There are normally a minimum of two drives for a system.

The printer on small systems is a character printer much like the typewriter. Most of these printers use a dot matrix or a typewriter print unit such as the daisy wheel.

There are different classifications used to separate the various kinds of computers. Figure 1 diagrams five system classifications.

System A—Pocket Computer

These units have just recently appeared in the market place. Ranging in price from $100 to $500, they have a full keyboard, a one-line display and are programmable in BASIC. The units can be interfaced with tape cassettes for off-line storage, to CRT displays, and to other systems via the telephone. Samples of the pocket computer currently include Radio Shack, Sharp, Panasonic, and Quasar. The market for these units is expected to soar in the 1980's (Goldfinger, 1980).

System B—Desk System

As the office of the future descends upon us, the terminal on every desk will be used more than the telephone. Typically, the subsystem will have its own processing capability with some disk storage. In remote locations the desk unit can tie to a central system periodically to transfer information back and forth. In a local environment it can be continuously connected to the office subsystem. A large amount of information will be stored and retrieved electronically as these systems become feasible. They will be used for communications, data collection, time management, reference to directories, and various word processing activities. Examples of the desk system include various intelligent terminals as well as computer units such as the Radio Shack models II and III,

Apple III, Commodore CBM, Xerox 820, and the Osborne. Prices range from $500 through $5,000. In the future, desk systems will normally cost under $500.

System C—Office System

There are close to a hundred suppliers of small business systems. Included in this class are the IBM 5120, Texas Instruments 990 series 4, DEC PDP11VO3, Datapoint 1800, Data General CS/20, and CADO system 40/IV. These systems can be configured for under $25,000. A system in this classification would be configured to handle a large percentage of the processing for an office. It would have a character printer and storage capacity for most of the current data used in the office.

FIGURE 1
SYSTEM CONFIGURATIONS

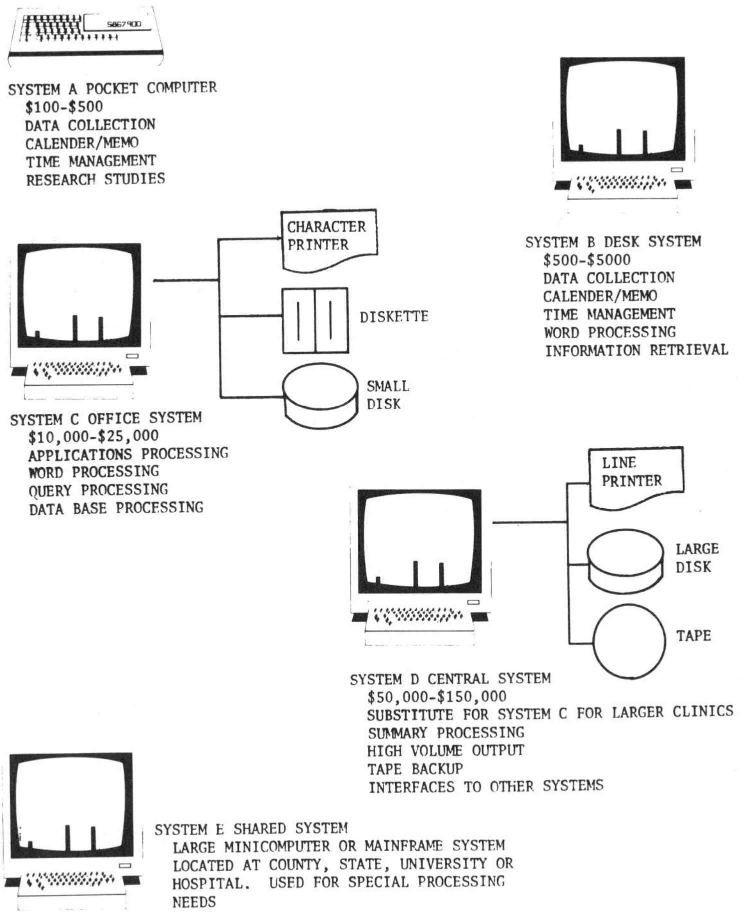

SYSTEM A POCKET COMPUTER
$100-$500
DATA COLLECTION
CALENDER/MEMO
TIME MANAGEMENT
RESEARCH STUDIES

CHARACTER PRINTER

DISKETTE

SMALL DISK

SYSTEM B DESK SYSTEM
$500-$5000
DATA COLLECTION
CALENDER/MEMO
TIME MANAGEMENT
WORD PROCESSING
INFORMATION RETRIEVAL

SYSTEM C OFFICE SYSTEM
$10,000-$25,000
APPLICATIONS PROCESSING
WORD PROCESSING
QUERY PROCESSING
DATA BASE PROCESSING

LINE PRINTER

LARGE DISK

TAPE

SYSTEM D CENTRAL SYSTEM
$50,000-$150,000
SUBSTITUTE FOR SYSTEM C FOR LARGER CLINICS
SUMMARY PROCESSING
HIGH VOLUME OUTPUT
TAPE BACKUP
INTERFACES TO OTHER SYSTEMS

SYSTEM E SHARED SYSTEM
LARGE MINICOMPUTER OR MAINFRAME SYSTEM
LOCATED AT COUNTY, STATE, UNIVERSITY OR
HOSPITAL. USED FOR SPECIAL PROCESSING
NEEDS

System D—Central System

The central system would be located regionally, or replace system C in larger urban organizations. This computer is a larger mini-computer based system in the range of $50,000 to $150,000. Examples of this system include the Texas Instruments 990, IBM system 34, PDP 11/34 and 11/45, WANG 2200, and Data General CS/40 and CS/60. These systems would typically handle all the processing requirements of the organization. There would still be communication links to other systems to transfer data.

System E—University, County, Hospital, or State Systems

These systems will continue to be used in a number of situations. Normally, these systems consist of larger main frames or larger mini-computers. They can be useful in situations where certain kinds of processing is necessary and the capability does not exist on the smaller system. They may also be used instead of system D as the central system. The difference is that system D would normally be dedicated to and under the control of the mental health unit, whereas system E would be shared with and controlled by the host user.

Potentials and Applications of Small Computers in Mental Health

Distributing Computer Power

The small computer is providing the means to distribute computing power to the point where it is needed at an economical cost. It will be used in conjunction with larger systems to provide the total computing needs of a mental health center. By the end of the 1980's the small computer will probably be providing 80% of the computing requirements of most community mental health centers. There will be a lot of emphasis on the automated office which includes word processing, electronic filing, and retrieval, electronic communication, and data processing. Systems will be linked together from the pocket computer through the small computer to other small computers or larger computers. Computer networks will be developed more extensively during the 1980's. Figure 2 shows some possible combinations of the systems described.

Combination 1 shows a single clinic using a small business system with terminals or desk units around the clinic. Interface with other systems is done through transferring data on diskettes. Combination 2 is the same as combination 1, but system D is used instead of system C. The size and volume of the organization requires the larger system, and there is no need for the ''C'' system. Combination 3 shows what is referred to in the industry as a hierarchical star network. This would be appropriate in an organization where there are a

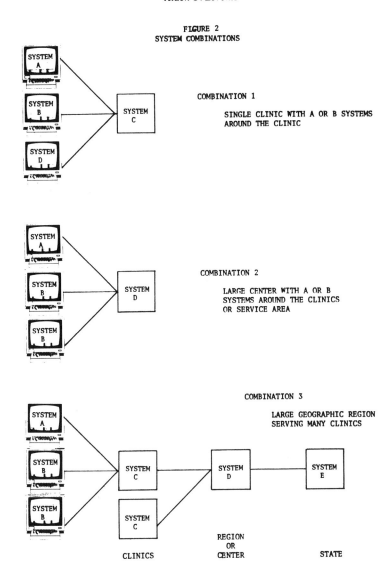

FIGURE 2
SYSTEM COMBINATIONS

COMBINATION 1

SINGLE CLINIC WITH A OR B SYSTEMS
AROUND THE CLINIC

COMBINATION 2

LARGE CENTER WITH A OR B
SYSTEMS AROUND THE CLINICS
OR SERVICE AREA

COMBINATION 3

LARGE GEOGRAPHIC REGION
SERVING MANY CLINICS

CLINICS   REGION OR CENTER   STATE

number of clinics served by an umbrella agency. These clinics are spread over a large geographic area. Local processing capability cuts down on online processing costs over long distances. This network configuration makes it possible to process centrally all data required centrally and allow local processing to be processed locally. It will also allow communication to be sent to all points from any other point through the central system.

Applications

System A (Pocket Computer) will have the potential of being used by clinicians in collecting data, assisting in time management, and maintaining memos. It also has the potential of gathering data while doing special studies on clients. The system can be tied in locally or remotely via telephone for transferring information either way.

System B (Desk System) is basically an intelligent terminal with some processing capability. It will be used by clincians and staff for the following tasks:

1. Display schedules
2. Retrieve client data
3. Enter data
4. Review client progress
5. Produce case notes
6. Enter and send correspondence
7. Reference directories
8. Memo/calendar functions

The processing capability of the desk system will allow staff the flexibility to use the units in various ways unique to their own operations.

The central office system (System C) will do about 80% of the processing for small clinics. This will include all financial processing, office of the future activities, and a large portion of the client and staff activity processing. The main restraint for system C will be the disk capacity, printer speed, and software capability. In larger clinics, system D will have to be used instead of system C. In other cases, system C will be used in conjunction with system D. The processing done on these systems will include most of the support necessary for the transaction processing and information requirements of a clinic.

These requirements can be categorized functionally as follows:

A. Clinical Care and Case Management
    1. Case Management
        a. Assessment
        b. Treatment Planning
        c. Treatment Monitoring
    2. Quality Assurance
    3. Clinical Record Keeping
        a. Client/Patient Information Categories
        b. Data Capture
        c. Organization and Scope of the Automated Client/Patient Record
B. Consultation and Education

C. Agency and Program Management
   1. Planning
       a. Identifying Catchment Area Needs
       b. Managing CMHC Programs
       c. Resource Allocation
   2. Financial Management
       a. Accounting
       b. Budgeting and Forecasting
       c. Cost-Finding
       d. Billing and Accounts Receivable
   3. Personnel and Manpower Management
       a. Personnel
       b. Labor Distribution
       c. Payroll
   4. Evaluation and Accountability
       a. Program Evaluation
       b. Accountability
D. Office Automation
   1. Document Creation
   2. Document Storage
   3. Communications
E. System Interfacing
   1. Federal Requirements
   2. State Requirements
   3. Local Requirements

The above functional requirements were taken primarily from the requirements statements as prepared by Libra Technology (Libra, 1980).

System E refers to large main frame systems located in other organizations such as universities, county or state government, and hospitals. These systems can be used to do the conversions necessary to interface the local system with other systems required by county, state, and federal programs. They can also be used to support statistical and processing requirements where software and processing capacity is lacking on the smaller systems.

Cautions Related to the Implementation of Small Computer Systems

The use of any computer system can create many problems. Many small businesses today are being lured into purchasing small computers like a typewriter or a copier. They do not realize that what they are purchasing is only the tip of the iceberg. The majority of the cost is in all of the other elements that go into making the system work. The hardware has in the recent past represented 60% of the total system cost. Today, hardware averages about 30% of the total cost, and it is expected to reach 10% of the total data processing budget in the 1980's. Figure 3 illustrates the iceberg effect of a computer system. The hardware is the part that is seen. The other elements contributing to costs either now or in the future are hidden.

Service, reliability, documentation, and system software are closely related to the hardware and are normally dependent upon the vendor. Many small systems have not been around long enough to establish a reliability track record. Service should be available within a reasonable distance at a cost that is in line with typical service costs. This can be a major problem in remote areas.

Documentation on how to use many systems is often incomplete, incorrect, written primarily for computer technicians, and not for the end users. The system software (operating system, editor, word processing package, languages) is not always friendly to the user. In other words, it takes a computer technician

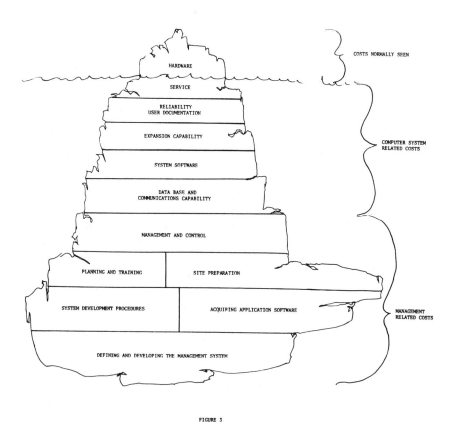

FIGURE 3

THE COMPUTER SYSTEM
ICEBERG

to understand it. The total system (hardware, software, applications, documentation) must be in harmony. If any portion of the system is weak the system becomes inoperable, and a great deal of money can be spent in trying to solve the problems.

The capability of the system is another dimension that can get the potential computer user in trouble. All systems should have communications capability to be able to communicate with other systems. Systems are often purchased to handle jobs that are beyond the capability of the system in terms of disk storage and printer speed. A major consideration must be expansion capability. If a new system is required in a couple of years to meet expanding requirements, it can be a costly process to change if the growth path has not been well planned.

There are other smaller items that tend to be forgotten in cost planning such as supplies, site preparation, space, and the training required to use both the computer system and the new data system. All individuals in the center are affected in some way.

To guard against getting into some of these traps, a detail cost plan should be developed that projects all costs related to the system over the next five years. Referencing an implementation guideline and preparing a checklist of budget items would uncover things that might be missed. A consultant may be helpful in developing this plan. It is better to spend the money on good plans rather than to spend it on getting out of trouble.

The larger cost items of the iceberg tend to be the definition of the management systems and the development of the application software (programming) to support these systems. Some of this can be acquired in package form, but normally there will be some modifications required to match the centers' systems with the package. Packages for client and event oriented data systems in mental health currently do not exist for the $10,000 to $25,000 computer systems. NIMH has developed, together with Libra Technology, a prototype design for an MIS to support CMHC's. It is intended that this design be converted to software that can be used on small computers. The documentation for this design is a good example of the effort required to define the management system, the information system requirements, and the software specifications necessary to implement a system. Hopefully, the results of this project will provide for many clinics around the country both design specifications and software. This will eliminate a duplication of high cost effort and make systems affordable where they may not now be possible.

Key elements in the development and distribution of a package that can be tailored to various centers are flexibility and standards. Flexibility can be achieved through the use of good database software design, report generators, and table driven applications. Standards tend to increase adaptability of the package to various brands of hardware and facilitate communication in using the package.

There are a number of turn key packages (hardware/software-combinations) on the market for CMHC's. Some of these systems are using state-of-the-art technology (database, report generators, screen generators, table driven software) making the packages flexible and user-oriented. These systems cost in the range of $70,000 to $150,000. This cost includes a considerable portion of the iceberg below the surface. However, there is still conversion, training, systems support, maintenance, and the ability to change to a new system to be considered.

Sources of Information Relating to Small Computers

The DATAPRO series is one of the most comprehensive sources for obtaining detailed information on every small computer available. DATAPRO also publishes reports on how to buy small systems and on who provides various software packages for these systems. A new volume has just been added that concentrates on small computers.

NIMH has published an excellent manual that is a planning and acquisition guide. The manual was authored by John A. Paton and Pamela K. D'huyvetter who were with Neoterics Inc. at the time. The two main sections include planning and designing the MIS and system acquisition and implementation.

The Minnesota Education Computing Consortium has done a good deal of experimenting with the use of the APPLE II for administrative use in school districts. This has been done in conjunction with central systems and communication links to distribute certain computing functions out to the school districts.

The project between NIMH and Libra Technology to develop a prototype MIS for community mental health centers promises to be a project with significant potential. The documentation is currently available in each of the state's mental health divisions. The continuation of this project has the potential for providing a package that can be useful to mental health centers across the country. This can reduce the high cost of centers having continually to develop their own systems. The documentation currently consists of the following documents.

1. Requirements Analysis
2. Suggested System Standard
3. Implementation Guide
4. System Design—Processing Logic
5. System Design—Data Content and Structure
6. Data Content and Structure—Appendix

Any center using computer systems or planning to increase this use of computer systems can obtain assistance from these documents. The implementation guide is extremely helpful for anyone considering system development or redevelopment. It is important to have an awareness of the various steps in the systems development cycle. Implementing systems does not begin with buying hardware and software. Sources referred to above and in the references can be very helpful in the development of a good implementation plan.

Summary

Small computers will have a significant impact on mental health centers during the 1980's. The continued advances in computer technology, together with price decreases, will provide affordable hardware even at the smallest centers. The challenges will be to provide the systems and the programs that will make this hardware adaptable to the needs of the centers. Center staff will need to become more cognizant of the problems and solutions toward implementing automated offices.

REFERENCES

Books

Billings, K., & Moursund, D. *Are you computer literate?* Portland, OR: Dilithium Press, 1979.
Brooks, F. P. *The mythical man-month.* Reading, MA: Addison-Wesley, 1975.
Cortada, J. W. *EDP costs and chances.* Englewood Cliffs, NJ: Prentice-Hall, 1980.
Couvey, D. H., & McAlister, N. *Computer consciousness: Surviving the-automated 80's.* Reading, MA: Addison-Wesley, 1980.
Paton, J. A., & D'huyvetter, P. K. *Automated MIS for mental health agencies: A Planning and acquisition guide.* NIMH. Washington, DC: U.S. Government Printing Office, 1980.
Sidowski, J. B., Johnson, J. N., & Williams, T. A. *Technology in mental health care delivery systems.* Norwood, NJ: Ablex, 1980.
Sipple, C. J., & Dahl, F. *Computer power for the small business.* Englewood Cliffs, NJ: Prentice-Hall, 1979.
Squire, E. *Introducing systems design.* Reading, MA: Addison-Wesley, 1980.

Studies

A feasibility study of administrative uses of microcomputers. Minnesota Educational Computing Consortium. 2520 Broadway Drive, St. Paul, MN 55113. May 1979.
Bellerby, L. *Survey of community mental health center information systems.* Regional Research Institute for Human Services. Portland, OR: Portland State University, 1980.
Goodman, J., & Wurster, C. *NIMH prototype management information system for community mental health centers.* Fourth annual symposium on computer applications in medical care. November 1980.
Hedlund, J., *et al. Mental health information systems: A state-of-the-art report.* Columbia, MO: University of Missouri, 1979.
NIMH prototype MIS community mental health centers. Five vols. Washington, DC: U.S. Government Printing Office, 1980.
1979–80 Microcomputer report. Minnesota Educational Computing Consortium, July 1979.

Periodicals

Byte, The Small Systems Journal. 70 Main St., Peterborough, NH 03458.
Computerworld. 375 Cochituate Rd., Route 30, Framingham, MA 01701.

Computers in Psychiatry/Psychology. 26 Trumbell St., New Haven, CT 06511.
Datamation. 666 Fifth Ave., New York, NY 10019.
Output. 666 Fifth Ave., New York, NY 10019.
Small Systems World. World Publishing, Inc., 53 W. Jackson St., Chicago, IL 60604.

Selected Journal Articles

Dowell, J. R. *So, you want to buy a minicomputer?* Price Waterhouse and Company Review, 1977.
Goldfinger, E. Office in a briefcase: Beyond the calculator. *Output,* June 1980.
Himrod, B. W. Microcomputers for small business. *Journal of Accountancy,* December 1979.
Howson, H. R. The microcomputer challenge. *CA Magazine,* August 1977.
Schoech, D. A microcomputer based human service information system. *Administration in Social Work,* Winter 1979.
Schwartz, D. A. Microcomputers take aim on small business clients. *Journal of Accountancy,* December 1979.

6. MANAGING FOR SUCCESS:
ASSESSING THE BALANCED
MIS ENVIRONMENT

Linda J. Bellerby, PhD
Lewis N. Goslin, PhD

This article reviews salient features involved in handling a management information system (MIS) support activity within a mental health agency. The significant points of the article follow. The major tasks of agency management of the information system are discussed. The general structure of MIS development and the MIS environment are presented. The conceptual features of assessment and balance of activities, including the macro dimensions for evaluating a system, are established. The attributes of macro dimensions as related to the stages of growth support the manager in determining an appropriate balance for a well-run MIS activity.

Agency Management of MIS

Agency management of automated management information systems (MIS) is not an easy task. The task can be even more difficult for the manager when it is not really clear what working balance is appropriate for the agency's MIS environment.

MIS is increasingly an area for interest by agency management. Two things are occurring. The use of MIS in mental health centers is increasing, and those existing "in-place" systems are becoming more sophisticated.

Dr. Bellerby is a Consultant, Nolan, Norton & Company, One Forbes Road, Lexington, MA 02173. Dr. Goslin is Professor, School of Business Administration, Portland State University, Portland, OR 97207. The research cited in this article was partially supported by a grant from the National Institute of Mental Health (Grant # 5 T24 MH 15446-01).

An increasing number of mental health managers are being confronted with the problems associated with developing an effective and efficient MIS. A 1979 survey of community mental health centers showed that 79 percent of the centers are using automated information systems (Bellerby, 1980). The majority of centers with manual information systems also had plans to automate within one year. In contrast, a 1974 survey reported that only 25 percent of the centers were using automated systems (Johnson, Giannetti, & Nelson, 1976). An obvious, dramatic observation is the increase in the number of centers using computers during the last five years.

MIS Development

An automated MIS for mental health agencies is composed of a set of computer applications which support critical agency activities. Such activities include:

—payroll
—billing
—clinical record keeping
—program evaluation
—staff activity accounting.

The effective implementation of these applications has to take into account how the system itself can modify conditions. Such modification due to the system can occur—within the agency organization itself, the technical dimensions of its programs, or in the management of individuals.

The relationship of the data processing function to other organizational units may need to be defined. New management techniques must be adopted to ensure that organizational resources are allocated and efficiently used to develop computer applications which provide the greatest benefit. Greater attention must also be given to understanding how the organization manages change or assesses the readiness to implement technological change through a balanced growth strategy. For the manager, the organizational, technical, and managerial aspects of MIS development must be taken into account.

MIS Environment

An important determinant of how well the agency's MIS environment is being managed is a simple assessment of the balance maintained among multiple aspects—macro dimensions—of information system development and operation. As an agency moves successfully to higher levels of management information system functioning, the growth of each of these macro dimensions must be coordinated and balanced against the capability of the agency to accept and support change in each area. The status of each dimension can be assessed with respect to its position on a growth continuum. Management attention can then be focused on dimensions which are out of balance. This assessment also helps managers prepare the transition of the agency for entry into the next stage of MIS growth.

Assessment and Balance

The manager with some experience in working with MIS development realizes that "fair" assessment and comparison is critical. Common sense says that a Jeep is not a Cadillac; a glass of grape juice is not wine; or a tangerine is not a grapefruit. Yet in *quick* comparative terms each of the prior mentioned pairs do possess many comparable attributes.

In the same way, comparing an agency's MIS development experiences with those in other mental health settings is risky unless the comparison is based on appropriate macro dimensions. A fair comparative assessment requires that the manager be aware what is the stage of development of the agency's MIS environment *and* what is the relative development of each macro dimension. For this comparison, the manager must know what is the MIS environment and what are appropriate macro dimensions. The critical issue then becomes: Is it possible to know? The answer is *yes* . . . within reasonable zones of balance.

Macro Dimensions

Community mental health centers (CMHCs) were studied and the macro dimensions of their information systems at different stages of growth were examined. The macro dimensions addressed by the study were:

— The set of computer applications;
— Management planning and control;
— User involvement strategies; and
— Organizational attitudes toward usefulness of the MIS.

These macro dimensions reflect the technical, managerial, and organizational behavior aspects of system development and provide the basis for assessing the degree of balance in the MIS environment. Viewing the MIS environment in this way is supported by earlier research which characterized the pattern of data processing growth in business organizations (Nolan, 1973; Gibson & Nolan, 1974; Nolan, 1979).

The study of CMHCs identified the key attributes of each macro dimension which distinguish among information systems at different stages of growth. Although these attributes do not represent an ideal model of information system growth, they are descriptive of typical attributes currently exhibited by mental health information systems at different stages of growth.

Attributes of Macro Dimensions

The study of the MIS environment in community mental health centers provides good insights for MIS managers. The study provides information about the attributes of the macro dimensions and how these attributes change. Evidence exists that:

—Distinct stages of information system growth can be characterized by profiles of computer applications common to community mental health centers in each stage. All of the centers studied could be classified into a designated stage.

—The profile of computer applications for centers in each stage shows that information system development generally progresses through incremental steps. These profiles provide an inventory of applications that reflect other managers' priorities for computer support.

—Increased formalization of management planning and control techniques is present for each stage of applications development. The areas where distinctions exist among stages include documentation of information handling procedures, charge-out for computer services, use of an information system steering committee, and assignment of information system priorities.

—User involvement strategies exhibit characteristics distinct for each stage of development. These characteristics show that centers develop more effective opportunities for user involvement in the system development process as they progress to more sophisticated uses of computer technology.

—Perceived usefulness and value is different at various stages of MIS growth. Centers which have developed the most comprehensive sets of computer applications reported the most favorable attitudes about their information system.

Determining the Stage

Determining the stage of growth of an agency's information system can be done by referring to Figure 1 which provides an assessment checklist of computer applications and Figure 3 which provides a checklist of attributes of management technique, user involvement, and organizational attitudes.

The checklist contained in Figure 1 contains three sets of computer applications which define the three distinct stages of information system growth found in CMHCs. Each set of applications is cumulative. For example, the applications which define Stage 3 represent the new applications which are implemented as an agency moves from Stage 2 into Stage 3.

Figure 1. CHECKLIST OF COMPUTER APPLICATIONS

Check YES or NO. The pattern of checks should
indicate stage of applications development.

STAGE	COMPUTER APPLICATIONS	YES	NO
1	Patient demographic characteristics	___	___
	Staff activity	___	___
	Intake data	___	___
	Direct service data	___	___
	Diagnostic data	___	___
	Indirect service data	___	___
OR			
	Patient demographic characteristics	___	___
	Third-party billing	___	___
	Direct patient billing	___	___
	Financial/accounting	___	___
	Payroll	___	___
	Staff activity	___	___
2	Patient demographic characteristics	___	___
	Third-party billing	___	___
	Direct patient billing	___	___
	Financial/accounting	___	___
	Payroll	___	___
	Staff activity data	___	___
	Intake data	___	___
	Direct service data	___	___
	Diagnostic data	___	___
	Indirect service data	___	___
3	Inventory system	___	___
	Cost outcome data	___	___
	Medication treatment plan	___	___
	Follow-up	___	___
	Utilization review	___	___
	Special symptom scales	___	___

Stage 1 is characterized by two distinct sets of applications. Centers in this stage either develop applications which support administrative functions such as payroll, accounting, and billing; or, they develop applications which support clinical record keeping functions through the automation of intake, direct and indirect service, and diagnostic data.

The set of applications for centers in Stage 2 is a composite of the two profiles which define Stage 1. In other words, centers in Stage 2 have developed a set of applications which support both administrative and clinical record keeping functions. The applications for Stage 3 reflect more emphasis on planning and evaluation.

A fourth grouping of applications also can be identified. These applications provide computer support for individual treatment plans, mental status examination, goal achievement data, clinical progress notes, development and social history, psychological screening, and clinical predictions. Although this set of applications may emerge as a potential fourth stage of applications development, few centers presently have operational computer support in these areas.

The procedure for determining an agency's stage of applications development is simple. Figure 1 can be used to record those applications where computer support is operational or under development. The distribution of applications across the three stages can then be assessed. Since agencies will not develop applications in precisely the sequence suggested by these stages, the following criteria provide the basis for a more realistic assessment: (1) the agency must have computer support operational or under development for *more than half* of the applications defined for the specified stage; and (2) computer support must be operational or under development for *more than half* of the applications defined for all preceding stages. An agency in Stage 1 will have computer support operational or under development for more than half of the applications included in one of the two profiles listed under that stage. Likewise, if an agency has computer support operational or under development for more than half of the applications listed under Stages 1, 2, and 3, the agency is in Stage 3 of applications development. Even if the set of applications developed by an agency does not entirely fit these criteria, a good idea of the approximate stage of development exists as compared to other community mental health centers. Figure 2 illustrates a typical profile of applications developed by a center classified in Stage 3 of development.

Figure 3 contains a set of attributes which will help assess an agency's stage of growth with respect to management planning and control techniques, user involvement strategies, and organizational attitudes toward the usefulness of the MIS. The study identified these attributes as being important in distinguishing among centers at different levels of information system growth.

These attributes can be evaluated by placing a check mark along the appropriate portion of the scale shown in Figure 3. The scale is partitioned into three sections which correspond to the three stages of applications development mentioned earlier. Figure 4 illustrates the status of each of these attributes for a center classified in Stage 3 of development.

Assessing the Balance

By comparing the pattern of responses in Figures 1 and 3, it is possible to assess the balance of the MIS environment. As responses are reviewed, too much attention should not be placed on any particular attribute. The attributes

Figure 2. CHECKLIST OF COMPUTER APPLICATIONS

EXAMPLE: CENTER WITH STAGE 3 APPLICATIONS

STAGE	COMPUTER APPLICATIONS	YES	NO
1	Patient demographic characteristics	X	
	Staff activity		X
	Intake data	X	
	Direct service data	X	
	Diagnostic data	X	
	Indirect service data	X	

OR ————————————————————

	COMPUTER APPLICATIONS	YES	NO
	Patient demographic characteristics	X	
	Third-party billing	X	
	Direct patient billing	X	
	Financial/accounting	X	
	Payroll	X	
	Staff activity		X

STAGE	COMPUTER APPLICATIONS	YES	NO
2	Patient demographic characteristics	X	
	Third-party billing	X	
	Direct patient billing	X	
	Financial/accounting	X	
	Payroll	X	
	Staff activity data		X
	Intake data	X	
	Direct service data	X	
	Diagnostic data	X	
	Indirect service data	X	

STAGE	COMPUTER APPLICATIONS	YES	NO
3	Inventory system	X	
	Cost outcome data	X	
	Medication treatment plan		X
	Follow-up	X	
	Utilization review	X	
	Special symptom scales		X

for each dimension are important in combination, not individually. In addition, the range presented for each attribute represents a general trend, a shift in the characteristics displayed by centers progressing to higher levels of MIS sophistication. How a specific agency makes this transition will vary. It is, therefore, not appropriate to expect every agency to display the precise characteristics designated along the portion of the scale corresponding to each stage. For example, not all centers in Stage 3 use formal criteria to establish system development priorities. These centers, however, are more likely to do so than centers classified in Stages 1 or 2. Since most of the Stage 3 centers have established an MIS steering committee, they are less likely to use informal

Figure 3.   CHECKLIST OF MACRO DIMENSION ATTRIBUTES

Check the portion of the scale that best describes your
agency.

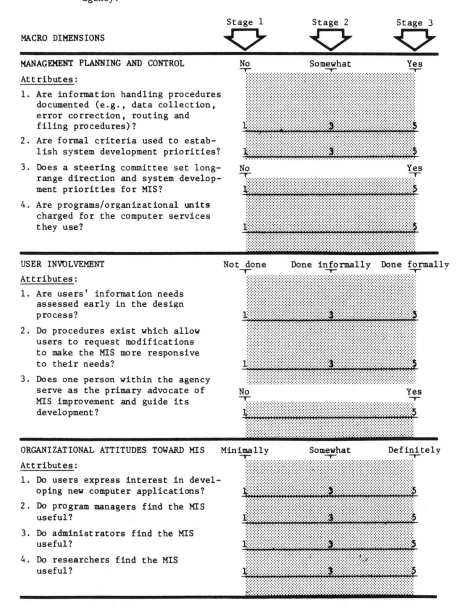

Figure 4. CHECKLIST OF MACRO DIMENSION ATTRIBUTES

EXAMPLE: CENTER WITH STAGE 3 APPLICATIONS

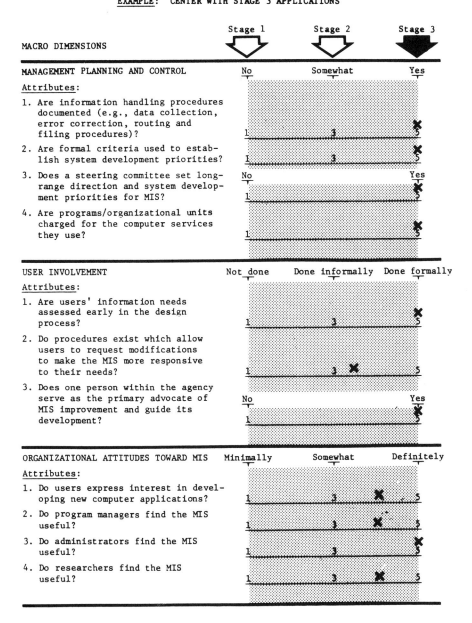

criteria, such as a first come, first served basis, for setting system development priorities.

If the responses in Figures 1 and 3 generally fall into the same stage, the MIS environment displays the type of balance common to CMHCs in the same stage of growth. The examples presented in Figures 2 and 4 illustrate this pattern.

Of greatest interest to managers are the macro dimensions with attributes consistently rated below the agency's present stage of applications development. Where responses display this pattern, those dimensions are identified which are out of balance relative to the technical sophistication of the MIS. Where improved MIS strategies may be needed, consideration of the MIS attributes of other centers in the same stage of applications development provide an evaluation framework for possible directions for change within the agency.

An example of an unbalanced MIS environment is illustrated in Figure 5. This profile of responses shows an agency in Stage 2 of applications development which has implemented no planning and control techniques or user involvement strategies. In this case, organizational attitudes would likely reflect user dissatisfaction with the MIS.

Where the attributes in Figure 3 were rated consistently higher than those commonly exhibited by centers at the same stage of applications development, the agency is probably in a good position to move to the next stage of MIS growth. This pattern of response is illustrated in Figure 6. In general, increased formalization of planning and control techniques and user involvement strategies reflects sound system development practices. Such development patterns can benefit agencies at any stage of growth.

Managing for Success

Astute managers realize that good management is both a science and an art. The management of MIS typifies this condition. The scientific aspect is most readily seen in the design of computer applications which effectively support critical agency activities. The art is reflected in making the best use of available resources and in integrating the experience and knowledge of users into the technical system design.

A manager's ability to merge successfully these two perspectives is facilitated by taking an integrated look at the MIS environment and recognizing the interrelationships that exist. The technical, managerial, and organizational behavior dimensions of MIS development must each be given fair consideration. Maintaining the appropriate balance requires managerial assessment of the relative stage of development of each dimension and managerial awareness of their future direction of growth.

Figure 5. CHECKLIST OF MACRO DIMENSION ATTRIBUTES

EXAMPLE: STAGE 2 APPLICATIONS/UNBALANCED MIS ENVIRONMENT

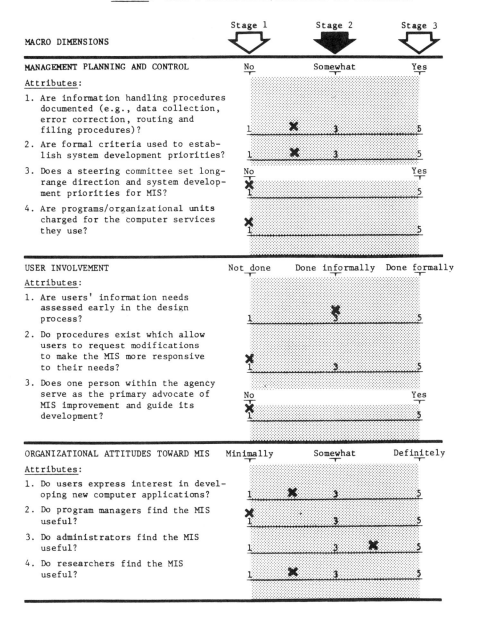

Figure 6.   CHECKLIST OF MACRO DIMENSION ATTRIBUTES

EXAMPLE: STAGE 2 APPLICATIONS/ADVANCED MIS ENVIRONMENT

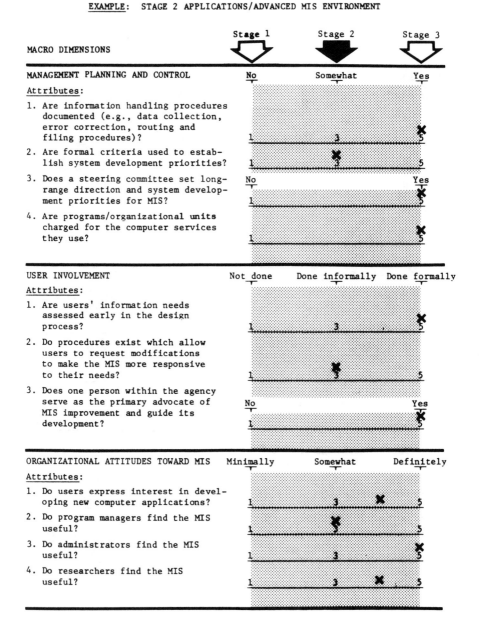

The astute manager of the MIS is aware of need, assessment, and dynamics. The manager is aware of the *need* for balance, the macro dimensions which *assess* the balance, and awareness necessitated by the *dynamics* of the organization, the system, and the people involved.

REFERENCES

Bellerby, L. J. *Patterns of information system growth in community mental health centers.* Unpublished doctoral dissertation, Portland State University, 1980.

Gibson, C. F., & Nolan, R. L. Managing the four stages of EDP growth. *Harvard Business Review*, 1974, *52*, 76–88.

Johnson, J. H., Giannetti, R. A., & Nelson, N. M. The results of a survey on the use of technology in mental health centers. *Hospital and Community Psychiatry*, 1976, *27*, 387–391.

Nolan, R. L. Managing the computer resource: A stage hypothesis. *Communications of the ACM*, 1973, *16*, 399–405.

Nolan, R. L. Managing the crises in data processing. *Harvard Business Review*, 1979, *57*, 115–126.

7. A DECISION SUPPORT SYSTEM
TO INCREASE EQUITY

Lawrence Boyd, Jr., PhD
Robert Pruger, DSW
Martin D. Chase, MSW
Marleen Clark, MSW
Leonard S. Miller, PhD

Every social service program faces the same basic question: *Which* clients should get *how much* of *what?* Here we suggest how a maintenance program (Miller & Pruger, 1975) could generate a continuously more equitable answer to that question. The central feature is a computer assisted Decision Support System (DSS) which informs the discretionary behavior of line workers, supervisors and managers (Keen & Morton, 1978; Alter, 1980).

Conventionally, equitable distribution is expected to result from a particular division of authority: high ranked officials produce regulations and guidelines; workers apply them to cases; and supervisors insure that worker applications are correct. Though these top down rules are regularly revised, they usually fail to achieve their fundamental intent—making consistent the critical decisions about clients made by line workers at the bottom. In the DSS described here that top down flow is reversed: programmatic wisdom moves from the bottom up.

Dr. Boyd is Visiting Associate Professor, Department of Political Science, Arizona State University, Tempe, AZ 85281. Dr. Pruger and Dr. Miller are Associate Professors, School of Social Welfare, University of California, Berkeley, CA 94720. Mr. Chase and Ms. Clark are Associate Specialists, Homemaker-Chore Project, School of Social Welfare, University of California, Berkeley. The demonstration project described in this article is funded by the Department of Social Services, State of California (Contract # DSS-CMB 38831).

The account that follows is based on our experience in designing and implementing such a system for the In Home Supportive Services Program (IHSS) in three California counties.

Top Down Decision Making in IHSS

IHSS is the single most expensive and one of the most controversial social service programs in California. It serves approximately 80,000 elderly, disabled clients at an annual cost approaching one-quarter of a billion dollars. Based on a legally prescribed home visit, the line worker makes two decisions about the client. First, he/she determines the client's degree of need (the worker's assessment decision). Second, he/she determines the weekly hours of service the client should receive (the worker's distribution decision) (Miller & Pruger, 1976). Both decisions are supposed to be guided by state and county regulations. These identify client disability groups and specify the kinds and maximum amounts of services that can be distributed to each.

In response to the rapidly rising cost of the program, regulations were regularly made more detailed. Workers had to allocate time across 30 or more discrete tasks (e.g., cleaning kitchen counters, sweeping, shopping, and the like), and different rules existed to guide each calculation. For example, with reference to bathroom cleaning, the maximum (under county guidelines) that could be awarded a client living alone in his/her own home was 20 minutes per week; if however, the client lived alone in a one-bedroom apartment, no more than 15 minutes could be awarded; and if the client lived with anyone over the age of 14, a maximum of 7.5 minutes could be granted.

With each cycle of rule revision, workers complained more bitterly about being reduced to low level accountants (Levy, 1970). And supervisors, of course, increasingly became the system's auditors. They served almost exclusively as conduits for passing along and doing the best they could to enforce regulations from the top. Most of their time was spent assuring that forms were properly filled out and that workers calculated service awards in a manner that conformed to the flood of regulatory criteria.

More than staff unhappiness was created, however. It became increasingly clear that the distribution of IHSS services was marked by substantial inequities: clients with the same degree of need received very different awards, and clients with very different degrees of need were awarded equal amounts of service (Miller & Pruger, 1977). More pointedly put, awards had less to do with client characteristics and more to do with the worker's ability to circumvent the established regulations. And many workers, for reasons given below, readily did so.

Rules are not self-implementing. What this means is that when workers do not accord legitimacy to the guidelines provided, they can, do, and will deviate from them (Hanlan, 1967). In place of a common standard, each worker more or less creates his or her own. Inequitable distribution is the inevitable result.

Workers provided us with a rich lore about the ease with which they ignored top down rules that violated their own informed appreciation of the client's predicament. They knew, for example, that a marginally higher award would pass undetected simply by awarding time for a task the client really did not need performed. And a substantially higher award could be made to appear to conform to the regulations simply by reporting an assessment that exaggerated the client's degree of disability.

Assessment and distribution rules created by officials distant from client and worker realities always will be vulnerable in this way. Hierarchically generated guidelines can create only the appearance of uniformity in the program. The accomplishment of uniformity in fact remains in the hands of the line workers, forever a function of how they choose to exercise the degree of discretion their jobs require them to have and which administratively cannot be withheld from them.

Workers will treat the collective wisdom of their peers as more authoritative or legitimate than that arising from any other source. Thus, they are most likely to voluntarily adjust their awards to bring them into greater conformance with the norms that are the essence of that wisdom. For these reasons the information system we designed had to be concerned with best ways to generate rules about clients awards from the bottom up.

To accomplish this a way had to be found to capture the collective wisdom of the workers and reflect it back to each one as he/she made decisions about clients. However, there were about 120 workers, and each had a more or less unique vision about what each kind of client ought receive. In addition, clients varied over many dimensions. Clearly, the usual "talking" methods (e.g., staff meetings, case conferences, in-service training) could not resolve this complexity. With the advent of the micro-computer (Schoech, 1979), however, the technological means existed for the requisite collaborative process to take place.

Design and Operation of the Decision Support System

Improving Assessment Decisions

In each IHSS district office we placed a microcomputer. It tells the worker the average number of hours all workers would award to a client of any given description. That average is based on what workers actually have awarded such a client over the recent history of the program. The more each worker, in determining any client's award, is guided by the same standards all workers are using, the more equity is advanced: like clients receive like awards no matter which worker actually handles the client's case.

In creating the system, the first task was to bring greater consistency to worker assessment decisions. Construction of client need scales began with a preliminary list of client characteristics that workers told us influenced their award decisions. That list included background characteristics, measures of physical functioning, socio-emotional functioning, and environmental factors, such as help from relatives. Data analysis reduced the resulting list of over 100 items by more than two-thirds, and from this came a set of quantitative client need scales to be used in calculating worker decision rules. Details of this data reduction process are contained in project documents (Miller & Pruger, 1977).

This initial process sparked sufficient dialogue between workers to yield an agreed upon, first edition of a standardized client assessment form. The form provided a means for reducing assessment inconsistencies and facilitated the entry of cases in the office microcomputers. Over time, both client need scales and client assessment forms continued to evolve through system feedback (Boyd, Miller, & Pruger, 1980).

Improving Distribution Decisions

As assessments became more reliable, it became possible to analyze worker distribution decisions to discover the implicit weights workers were, on average, giving to different disability factors in determining client awards. This analysis resulted in a distributive formula or algorithm which, once entered into the computer, would convert a worker's assessment of a client into a predicted award.

To understand better the origin and role of the distributive rule formula, imagine that the only connection of importance was between hours awarded and a single need factor. This connection can be summarized in the simple linear equation,

$$H = bN + e.$$

In this formula, H stands for the number of hours per week awarded each client; N represents the need level for each client; b is the weight workers, on average, assign to the need factor; and e is the amount in hours not predicted by the need factor for each client. The value of b is mathematically estimated from all the workers' decisions. If that value is 4, then the computer would subsequently predict an additional four hours of service for each unit increase in the need factor. For example, a client with a need score of 5 would get a computer prediction of $4 \times 5 = 20$ hours of service per week.

Measuring Equity

Given the distributive rule formulas, it became possible to report how much workers strayed from current collective wisdom. That information is contained in the e term of the distributive formula. One such measure is the *average* amount that all workers deviated from the hours predicted by the distributive rule formulas. Another is the statistical index of prediction consistency known as R-squared. That measure runs from 0, for absolute inconsistency, to 1, for perfect consistency. This information is essential for evaluating how well programs are producing equity. For example, an office with an average miss of 6 hours is doing less well than an office missing by 4 hours, and an office with an R-square value of .6 is doing less well than an office with a value of .8.

System Cycles and Feedback

Given the complexity of clients' needs and other factors, distributive rule formulas are much more complex than described above. Therefore, the system was designed to evolve toward greater realism and precision through successive approximations and feedback. The process proceeds through the following steps:

1. Workers enter assessment information for each client into the microcomputer;

2. On the microcomputer screen workers receive the prediction from the previously identified distributive rule formula advising them of what all other workers would have awarded a client of like description. The prediction is not a command. It is merely information to the worker to guide the exercise of his or her discretion (Inbar, 1979);

3. Should a worker's award be substantially higher or lower than the prediction, the worker is prompted for a comment on the uniqueness of that case. The comment (e.g., "Must see doctor 3 times per week and no public transportation is available"; "Client is very independent, refuses some of the service hours offered") is entered into and stored in the computer;

4. Cases accumulated during the current cycle (approximately a three month period) are analyzed to update the distributive rule formula;

5. Observed deviations and worker comments are analyzed to discover potentially relevant new criteria regarding clients and program considerations;

6. Unit meetings are held for workers to review their reports, discuss their comments, and provide feedback;

7. Worker assessment forms and the computer program are revised to reflect changes in criteria; the refined distributive rule formula is put in the computer program; and the next cycle begins with step one.

The Reporting Function

The analysis done in each cycle results in a set of computer generated reports that are distributed to the workers. Selected reports are shown in Figures 1–5. The center vertical line in those figures represents the predicted average award for a given client. Each asterisk, representing the worker's actual decisions, shows the deviation of the worker's award from the predicted award. The actual amount of deviation in hours can be read on the horizontal axis of the graph. Cases are ordered on the graph according to number of hours predicted, increasing from top to bottom.

The worker report contained in Figure 1 is a portrait of inequity. The decisions observed there are inconsistent in terms of what all other workers on the average would have decided. They are internally inconsistent as well since clients with the same need were given very different amounts of service. Here is a worker who ignored the information system altogether and who, through incompetence or inexperience, has treated clients inequitably.

Figure 2 presents another very undesirable decision profile. With virtually every case falling on the prediction line, it is clear that this worker entirely relinquished discretionary responsibility to the client. In addition, the learning capacity of the system depends on the detection of departures from what the system knows about distributive behavior at any point in time. The forfeiting of worker discretion is especially serious in early cycles of system development.

Figure 3 shows the more ideal decision pattern. Some scatter about the prediction line reflects expected imprecision in the system or the worker and

Figure 1.   Award pattern of worker applying no consistent set of
            distributive rules.

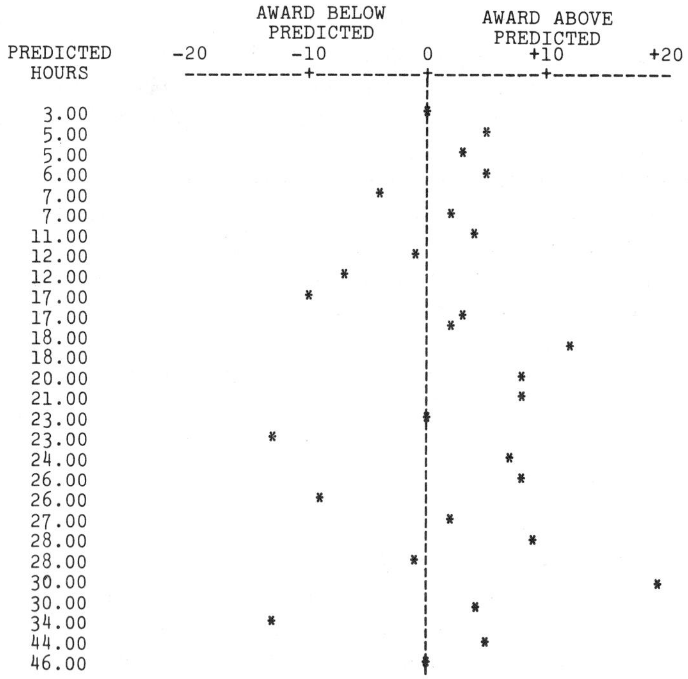

Figure 2.   Award pattern of worker not using discretionary
            judgment.

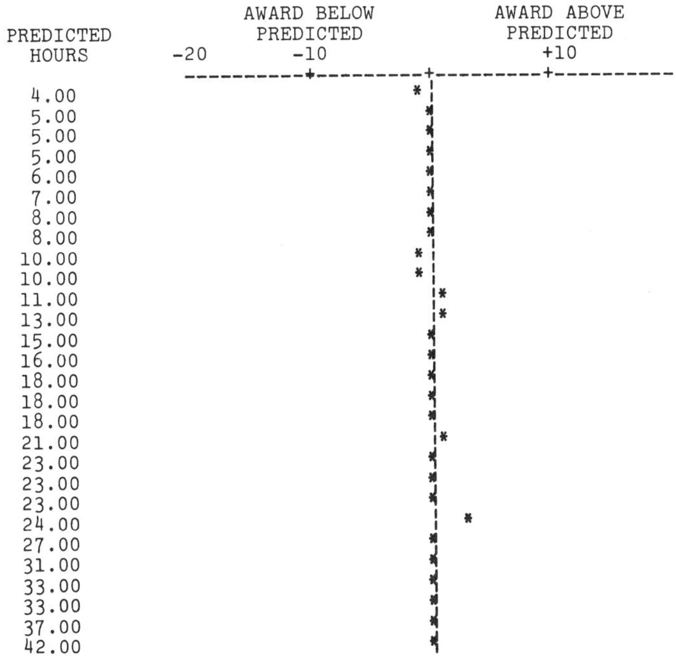

```
                       AWARD BELOW          AWARD ABOVE
   PREDICTED            PREDICTED            PREDICTED
    HOURS       -20       -10                  +10
              ----------+---------+---------+----------
     4.00                              * |
     5.00                                |*
     5.00                                *|
     5.00                                *|
     6.00                                *|
     7.00                                *|
     8.00                                *|
     8.00                               *|*
    10.00                            *   |
    10.00                            *   |
    11.00                                |*
    13.00                                |*
    15.00                                *|
    16.00                                *|
    18.00                                *|
    18.00                                *|
    18.00                                |*
    21.00                                |*
    23.00                                *|
    23.00                                *|
    23.00                                *|
    24.00                                |    *
    27.00                                *|
    31.00                                *|
    33.00                                *|
    33.00                                *|
    37.00                                *|
    42.00                                *|
```

the fact that the worker was exercising discretion. The two observations falling
far outside the normal range of cases have very special significance. They
might reflect very serious worker errors. However, given the overall portrait of
a competent, conscientious worker, they more likely provide evidence of
relevant information unrecognized by the system. That information is requested by the computer upon entering the case.

Figures 4 and 5 are included to suggest how much more about the implicit
distributive rules of individual workers can be observed in the worker reports.
The distinctive pattern of the conscientious, competent worker is observed in
both instances. The difference is that these two workers are not applying the
same decision rules as the majority of workers.

Figure 4 shows a worker consistently giving more than other workers, on
the average, would have given.

Figure 5 depicts a worker who consistently gives less to clients who are
relatively low on need and gives more to clients who are higher on need than
other workers on average would have given.

The two workers represented in Figures 4 and 5 have very different ideas
about how awards should be made. In addition, both their philosophies differ

Figure 3.   Award pattern of worker distributing in accord with
            existing normative rules.

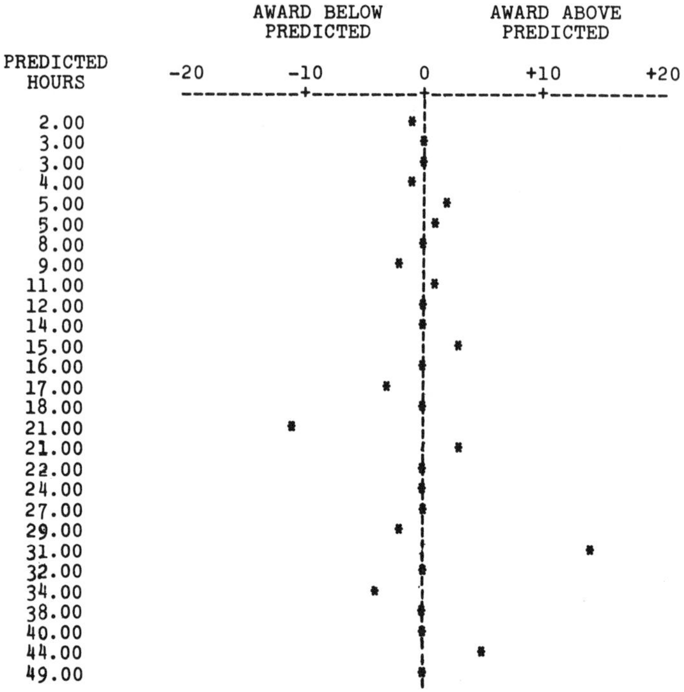

```
                    AWARD BELOW              AWARD ABOVE
                    PREDICTED                PREDICTED
     PREDICTED
      HOURS      -20        -10        0        +10        +20
                 ----------+---------+---------+----------
      2.00                                *|
      3.00                                *|
      3.00                                 |
      4.00                                *|
      5.00                                 | *
      5.00                                 |*
      8.00                                 *
      9.00                             *   |
     11.00                                 |*
     12.00                                 *
     14.00                                 *
     15.00                                 |  *
     16.00                                 *
     17.00                          *      *
     18.00                                 *
     21.00                *                 |
     21.00                                 |  *
     22.00                                 *
     24.00                                 *
     27.00                                 *
     29.00                         *       |
     31.00                                 |             *
     32.00                                 *
     34.00                           *     |
     38.00                                 *
     40.00                                 *
     44.00                                 |   *
     49.00                                 *
```

markedly from that of the majority of workers. Yet these deviant perspectives
clearly are worthy of attention. An important function of the system is that it
facilitates rational, focused arguments about such differences. Nevertheless,
as long as any workers are operating on different decision rules, clients are not
being treated equitably.

As the information system developed, additional kinds of reports for workers were produced. Among other things, these reports tell each worker how the
pattern of his/her assessment and distribution decisions compares to the pattern of his or her unit and county, including notation and interpretation where
significant differences occur. Various aggregations of worker reports are
prepared for supervisors and managers.

Implementation and Performance of the DSS

The initial reaction of workers to the Project ran from apathy to hostility. Of
approximately 120 workers, no more than twelve to fifteen welcomed it. Most
saw the Project as simply another tool of administration to eliminate the
worker's job, reduce its discretionary content, or generally harass those on the

bottom. For others, it was the next step toward the dehumanization of the welfare client. A miscellaneous category of complaints included accusations of a Marxist plot; claims that the only benefit would be several more doctoral dissertations; and even the unanswerable query:

How do we know that you won't come into the building when it's closed and put a lower prediction into the computer so that we're gradually forced to lower our awards?

We decided to cultivate the most positive workers and allow enough time to pass for the others to discover for themselves that their fears were groundless: jobs were not lost, worker discretion increased, accountant-like job content and paper work was much reduced, deviance from the prediction not only was not punished but actually was used to improve the prediction, and the like. Only a small number of workers achieved a working understanding of how the distributive formula was computed and changed, though the opportunity was offered to all. But even the least knowledgeable worker increasingly could not deny what he/she experienced: over time the computer prediction for any client

Figure 4. Award pattern of worker consistently over-awarding in comparison to normative rules.

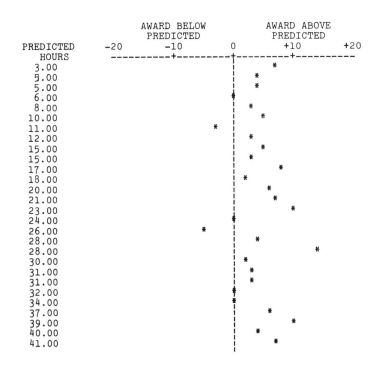

Figure 5.   Award pattern of worker reducing normative awards at lower
            disability levels; increasing normative awards at higher
            disability levels.

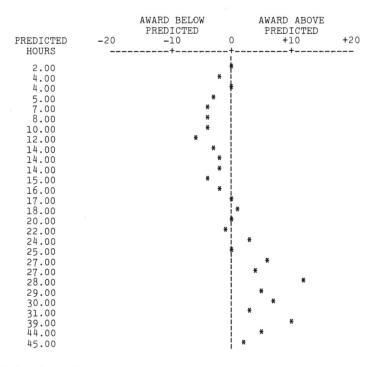

and what the worker independently thought ought to be awarded to that client got closer and closer.

Our implementation strategy also had to take into account the welfare system's deeply embedded orientation to top down decision making. Though workers endlessly ridiculed and routinely deviated from rules that came from above, they were not necessarily ready, willing, and able to cooperate with each other to create their own rules. And many supervisors were quite comfortable with their auditor's role. They knew how to check on workers and they had the agency's support for doing so. On both counts they harbored real doubts about the Project's encouragement to become leaders instead of auditors.

In such an environment, the attitudes, skills, and behaviors required by bottom up decision making could be learned, if at all, only at a very measured pace. We decided, therefore, to expand the degree of collaboration needed very slowly. Thus, in the first phase of the Project the achievement of equity was attempted only at the office level. The hope was that all actors would learn to meet the requirements of more complex levels of cooperation by first facing and solving problems that arose at less complex levels. As circumstances justified it, our efforts turned to the creation of equity within increasingly larger administrative units—the district division, the entire county, and currently, the multiple county grouping.

When the project began approximately 60% of the variance in client awards was explained by variance in client characteristics. Today, almost two years later, that figure is up to 85% and is still rising. Thus, the 120 workers in the three demonstration counties, many of whom never see or speak to each other, appear to be following the same rules and applying them with a very high degree of consistency. At the heart of this achievement is microcomputer technology. It made it possible for these workers for the first time to have the information their discretionary decisions required. Once so informed, equity increased even in the context of many fewer top down rules and less hierarchical oversight.

Ingredients of a Successful Information System

It should surprise no one that every element of the design, implementation, and performance of the DSS described above was more complicated than our account might have implied. We have emphasized the "success" of the system because the literature is replete with descriptions and analyses of failure (Wildavsky, 1980). Much more is known about why information systems do not work than how they might work better. This paper concludes with a summary of the major features of the equity oriented DSS that have contributed to its success.

Phased Implementation

Implementation of the DSS all at once could only have resulted in a disaster: systems can learn only at a certain rate. The wisest strategic choice we made was to introduce the DSS slowly. This had many productive applications, including the following:

a. As already mentioned, equity was first sought at the office level and only slowly expanded to successively larger administrative jurisdictions. Thus, in smaller offices, each worker had to reconcile his/her vision of "which client ought get how much of what" with only seven others. Once some comfort with that process had been achieved, and the requirements of equity were better understood, reconciliation at more complex levels could be attempted.

b. Only one thing *had* to happen in order for the computer prediction to get better over time: workers had to enter all their cases into the computer, give the award they thought was most justified, and enter a comment when the award and prediction differed substantially. Consequently, all our efforts in the first year were directed toward getting this to occur. Other than attending to ceremonial requirements or securing the easily obtained permissions needed, we essentially ignored the supervisors and managers. We knew that the role of these higher ranked officials would ultimately have to be changed in a fully operating DSS, but we muted these considerations until the more essential, minimal degree of worker cooperation had been achieved. Confidence, as well as rules, was to be created from the bottom up.

c. When the Project began we consciously programmed the computer to ask for an explanation only when the difference between the predicted and actual award was so large that very few workers would be asked for a comment. This had two great advantages. First, the initial interaction between the large majority of workers and the computer was positive. That is, the computer implicitly conveyed to these workers that their award decisions were equitable. Second, the few worker decisions that were challenged had such clearly deviant elements that it was relatively easy either to categorize the decision as inequitable or use it to improve the distributive formula. As worker confidence grew and the formula improved, the range of deviance that was unquestioned was made narrower.

Minimizing Costs and Risks for DSS Users

Eliciting support for the DSS requires persistent efforts to minimize the costs and risks and increase the benefits perceived by each actor as being associated with its use. This insight had applications such as the following:

a. The DSS resulted in an intake form that was much shorter than workers previously had to use. Even for those workers who still do not understand or care about either the DSS or increasing equity, the shorter form has been sufficient reason for them to voluntarily continue their essential degree of participation. Probably no single cost reducing step we took has been so productive.

b. If the distributive formula was to improve, workers had to feel free to deviate from the computer prediction when their knowledge of the client warranted it. Many workers, however, balked on the grounds that their supervisors would take the computer prediction as the correct standard and, in one way or another, would penalize workers who deviated from it. To calm these fears we arranged to have supervisors officially told that they were in neither overt nor subtle ways to reward or punish workers for any use they might make of the prediction. We never really knew whether worker fears were justified or not. Nevertheless, they had to be taken seriously because they were real in the workers' minds.

c. Regular efforts were made to minimize the time it took for the worker to enter a case into the computer and get a prediction from it. (Currently, this takes about two minutes.) In addition, the format of the computer program (which the worker experiences as an ordered set of questions that appear on the computer TV screen), was continuously made more flexible as workers indicated the need for it. This included such things as making it very easy to correct or change a previous entry. To encourage workers to weigh the prediction carefully, the format was adjusted to enable workers to enter their assessment, receive a prediction, and return to the computer at a later time to enter their award without having to reenter the information about that case.

 d. Until sufficient confidence developed, workers used both the prediction and the program's traditional time per task criteria to determine client awards. This enabled each worker to try the new methodology to the extent he or she felt comfortable with it. In addition, it minimized the fears of supervisors and managers that worker generated rules would result in chaos and/or substantial budget shortfalls. While the use of parallel regulatory systems may seem awkward, it made it much easier for those at all hierarchical levels to allow something new to be tried.

Research Capability

 Even with a great deal of worker cooperation, the distributive formula never would have gotten any better if the Project lacked a strong research capability. Substantial technological expertise was employed to produce better and better models of worker decision behavior. This, in turn, led to distributive formulas that yielded predictions that became increasingly credible in the eyes of the workers. In the absence of this analytic capability, no other combination of Project properties would have been sufficient to create and sustain worker confidence.

 The design and operation of a successful DSS requires a rare combination of technological, program, and human relationship skills. As a well funded, politically supported, university based demonstration project, we were able to put this combination together. But it is less likely that a public social service agency, with its normal staff complement and workload, could. Thus, the question is: could such an agency operate the kind of DSS described here on its own? In our case, at least, we will soon know. The final Project year, which is just beginning, is to be devoted to training line and staff personnel at all hierarchical levels for their roles in an entirely agency operated, equity oriented information system. Our expectation is that the needed technical expertise probably can be created. We are less certain that the skills and attitudes that support intra- and inter-rank cooperation, and which keep the information system fresh and dynamic, can be developed. But that uncertainty is preferable to the certain disappearance of the DSS if the Project ended merely with a report to the participating agencies that fully explained and documented the "success' described in ths paper.

REFERENCES

Alter, S. *Decision support systems: Current practice and continuing challenges*. Reading, MA: Addison-Wesley, 1980.

Boyd, L., Miller, L., & Pruger, R. *Equity and efficiency project: First year report*. Berkeley: School of Social Welfare, University of California, 1980.

Hanlan, A. Counteracting problems of bureaucracy in public welfare. *Social Work*, 1976, *12*, 88–94.

Inbar, M. *Routine decision making: The future of bureaucracy*. Beverly Hills: Sage Publications, 1979.

Keen, P., & Morton, M. S. *Decision support systems: An organizational perspective*. Reading, MA: Addison-Wesley, 1980.

Levy, G. "Acute" workers in a welfare bureaucracy. In D. Offenbacher & C. Poster (Eds.), *Social problems and social policy*. New York: Appleton-Century-Crofts, 1970.

Miller, L., & Pruger, R. *The division of labor in a perfect maintenance agency*. Berkeley: School of Social Welfare, University of California, 1976.

Miller, L., & Pruger, R. *Final report of the homemaker-chore study*. Berkeley: School of Social Welfare, University of California, 1977.

Miller, L., & Pruger, R. *The two activities of social services: Maintenance and people changing*. Berkeley: School of Social Welfare, University of California, 1975.

Schoech, D. A microcomputer based human services information system. *Administration in Social Work*, 1979, *3*, 423–440.

Wildavsky, A. *Information as an organizational problem*. 1980 (mimeographed).

8. COMPUTERIZING AN INTEGRATED CLINICAL AND FINANCIAL RECORD SYSTEM IN A CMHC: A PILOT PROJECT

Jim Newkham, ACSW
Leon Bawcom, MS

Today is the age of accountability; at the very least, that means the public has the right to know what it is spending its money for and that the money is being spent appropriately and effectively. According to Schoeck and Arangio (1979), ''the human service field is moving toward increased accountability and sound management.'' Accountability requires effective management with a clear idea of who is to be served and at what cost. In addition, the services must be of high quality and efficiently delivered. It is increasingly difficult for human service agencies to maintain financial data, clinical records, and effectively serve clients.

Automation is a viable option to meet these demands effectively, especially for an MHMR center such as ours. This is a description of the Heart of Texas Region Mental Health Mental Retardation (HOTRMHMR) Center's three-year experience in developing and implementing an automated Staff/Management Information System (S/MIS).

The Heart of Texas Region MHMR Center in Waco is a quasi-governmental, full service mental health and mental retardation center providing inpatient, outpatient, drug abuse, geriatric, regional, children, 24-hour, and day/evening care services for MH and MR clients through 15 service locations. The Center

Mr. Newkham is Director of Outpatient Services, and Mr. Bawcom is Director of Crisis Intervention Services, Heart of Texas Region Mental Health and Mental Retardation Center, P.O. Box 1277, Waco, TX 76703.

serves a six-county region with a population of 258,000 persons in both urban and rural areas. Annually, 5,000 persons are screened and 2,700 persons are served in one or more of the above programs. Of 126 staff, 14% are administrative with some direct service responsibility, 63% clinical with total direct service responsibility, and 23% are support staff. The budget was $2.8 million for the fiscal year ending August 31, 1981. The Center's service delivery system is tied to many other agencies, local and state-wide, through follow-up of state facility patients, aging services, child protective programs for neglected and abused children, the criminal justice system, area health agencies, area planning agencies, and other mental health and retardation programs.

When the Center's administrative staff examined the agency's clinical and financial operations in 1976, it found the information system lacking in the following areas: (1) turn-around time was four to six months before receiving data back from the state MHMR office; (2) when received, there was little trust in the accuracy of the data; (3) factual data or knowledge of active and inactive caseloads and knowledge of staff and client service data was essentially unavailable to direct service staff or management; (4) manual tracking and reporting systems including revenue and expenditure data was time consuming and did not provide detail information necessary for accountability to funding sources; (5) case records were non-standardized, disorganized, and summary clinical information could not be readily obtained; (6) maintaining audit standards was difficult and laborious due to the unaccessibility of needed data; and (7) cost outcome analysis was primitive and essentially non-existent.

The first priority addressed in solving these problems was the cleaning up of our data reporting system to the state. This was accomplished through restructuring the methodology and monitoring of the reporting data prior to forwarding. The second step was standardizing our clinical records system in order to become auditable from a clinical point of view. Improvement of the financial system was critical as the agency was, at that time, dealing with a $110,000 deficit. Thus, staff began exploration of computer service bureaus, seeking automation capabilities that could satisfy the multiple clinical and financial reporting demands. Due to the success in significantly reducing errors in our manual reporting system, we were recommended by Dr. Jack Franklin of the Texas Department of MHMR and the audit staff of Texas Department of Human Resources to develop a pilot automated system. The state agencies were interested in a system being developed to provide a viable audit trail for services and reimbursement and to examine the feasibility of operating a comprehensive data system in a community mental health center and transmitting its reporting data via computer tapes.

The Center's goal was to develop an automated information system that would assist in improving and maintaining the quality of services while resolving the standards compliance issues involved in accountability. The major objectives necessary to reach the above stated goals included the development of: (1) a Problem Oriented Record (POR); (2) an effective data collection process; (3) an automated fiscal reporting system; and (4) a computer hardware and software system. The Texas Department of Human Resources agreed to fund the software develoment, and the Center agreed to purchase the hardware, fund the maintenance of the hardware, and commit itself to the development of the Staff/Management Information System.

Implementation Philosophy

With funding secured to develop an automated records system, the Center staff felt that several key management principles were central to the successful development of this system. Although there are many management styles in use today, the one selected was one of Enabling rather than one of Controlling. The Enabling style of management relies heavily on (1) multi-level staff being actually involved in the decision-making process, (2) the idea that the combined action or product of a group of people (Synergy concept) produces more effective decisions, and (3) people want to do the best job they can, given the information and resources needed to complete the job.

This meant all levels of staff would be involved in the design of the system from the very beginning and would be given real decision-making authority, not a token involvement. In addition, there would be enough concern and confusion when introducing an impersonal communication tool, like a computer, into a human service delivery system without management being perceived as having ulterior motives towards its use. Hence, genuine and continuous involvement of staff from data clerks, front line clinicians, support staff, unit and program directors, top administrators, and the governing board was planned to facilitate internal support and cooperation as the bedrock upon which to develop the automated system.

A second management principle was the issue of a staff information system vs. a management information system. A staff information system is any method by which staff gathers, stores, processes, evaluates, and presents information about a particular client or group of clients and in turn is used by staff to monitor, evaluate, and make decisions concerning that client or group of clients. A management information system is any method by which an organization gathers, stores, processes, evaluates, and presents information which then is used by management to monitor, evaluate, and make decisions concerning the organization. Past experience with an imposed data system led the HOTRMHMR to plan for a staff information system which gave immediate feedback to all levels of staff who were putting data into the system, with management information as a by-product. Therefore, the term Staff/Management Information System (S/MIS) was coined to describe the system.

A third important management principle was to provide through the S/MIS accurate, cohesive information, not just unrelated data. Data is simply facts, whereas information is facts compiled and related in ways that have meaning to staff involved and communicates knowledge for effective decision-making. Useful information allows one to monitor, plan, and compare progress toward the goals of the system, from the front line clinician to the top level administrator. For the system to function effectively, the information must be readily accessible, timely, and easily understood, and having common definitions which can be summarized for comparison and related to the goals or purposes of the service system.

The last principle considered important to the system's success was simplicity. The amount of data available for computerization in a medium-sized community mental health center such as the HOTRMHMR can be overwhelming. A seductive feature of an automated system is the assumed capability to obtain data about everything in several different ways; however, a practical approach toward simplicity with as little paperwork as possible was adhered to in developing the system remembering the old adage "keep it simple."

From the inception and planning for this project, the enabling management concept was central, with practicality and common sense being the touchstones in developing the data components into the integrated Staff/Management Information System.

The Implementation Process

Actual implementation began with the management staff determining the four major components to be considered in designing the automated system. These components included the software development, the hardware system, the state mental health data system, and the local community mental health center system. The first step was to select a software consultation group. The primary reason for selecting the software company was their past experience with other mental health information systems. The agreement with the software group called for their working with the center staff in the design, development, and de-bugging of the automated system with the contractual cost for software development of $154,000.

The hardware configuration selected, with consultation by the software company, was a Wang 2200 VS which included core memory of 256K and 75 million characters of disk storage, one 600-line-per-minute printer, one 9-track tape drive, and four CRT work stations. This configuration was felt, at the time, to be the most cost-effective system on the market and the most compatible system for the amount of data a mid-sized center would process. The hardware cost was $69,000 with a yearly maintenance cost of $12,600.

Work with the state mental health data system involved a change from sending manual forms, which were batched and mailed in bulk to the state office, to sending a magnetic tape with summarized service data. The negotiations focused on the complicated process of deciding and agreeing on exactly what data was to be sent within a format which would allow the state computer to receive the Center's data and incorporate it into the overall state data collection process. By necessity, the phase was lengthy and complicated and involved discussions among the Center, the software group, and the state MHMR data staff.

Within the agency, the system's development involved all levels of staff providing input into the process with specific responsibilities defined. The Director of Support Services was charged with the development of forms to provide both hard copy for the clinical records and input documents for the computer; the Director of Finance was charged with the automation of the financial system; and the Problem Oriented Record (POR) Committee composed of clerical, clinical, and administrative staff was charged with the development of the automated clinical system. The Executive Director played the pivotal role of settling issues and questions and enabling negotiations among the groups.

A review of the literature for models of integrated automated information systems provided little in the way of assistance. However, there were sources helpful in providing guidelines (Meldman et al., 1976; Newman et al., 1978; Newman & Sorensen, 1981). The system had to be designed to meet a number of criteria: (1) it had to be supportive of the client flow through the Center's treatment process with a minimum of paperwork, yet capture accurate data and provide documentation of services; (2) it had to be helpful to the direct service provider by giving immediate feedback to help keep records current; (3) it had to meet the reporting needs for client and service data; (4) it had to meet the financial reporting requirements for the Center's numerous funding sources and provide an audit trail for fiscal review; (5) it had to provide summary information for client and system management; and (6) it had to lend itself to cost outcome analysis.

As noted earlier, the existing record system of the Center was nonstandardized; thus in converting to the automated problem oriented record system, a completely new record system was designed to meet these criteria. The formalization of this process began by laying out each important step of the client's flow through the system from screening and clinical history development to the discharge summary. The POR Committee, working in conjunction with the Director of Support Services, designed and developed each form to capture specific client data at each major treatment juncture. (See Table 1.) A multisection folder, with a record organization and content procedure, was used to organize the clinical record material.

Contact and Intake Forms were developed to provide the basic demographic data base for input into the computer. A Level of Functioning Scale (LOF) was designed, based on the work of Newman (1978), as a brief rating scale of a person's ability to function independently. A Master Problem List was developed corresponding to the nine areas of functioning on the LOF in order to

Table 1
CLIENT FLOW AND DOCUMENTATION PROCESS

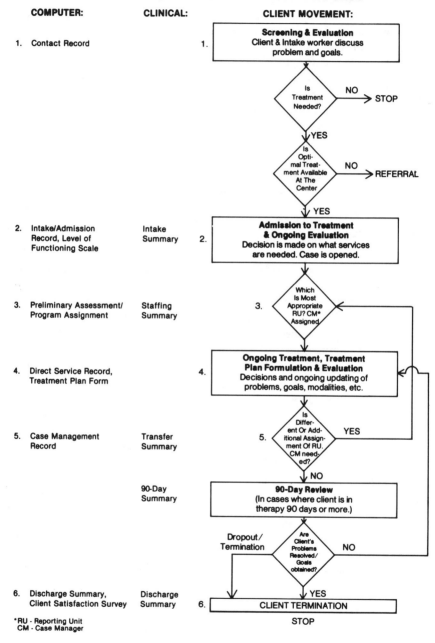

COMPUTER:

1. Contact Record
2. Intake/Admission Record, Level of Functioning Scale
3. Preliminary Assessment/ Program Assignment
4. Direct Service Record, Treatment Plan Form
5. Case Management Record
6. Discharge Summary, Client Satisfaction Survey

*RU - Reporting Unit
CM - Case Manager

CLINICAL:

Intake Summary
Staffing Summary
Transfer Summary
90-Day Summary
Discharge Summary

CLIENT MOVEMENT:

1. **Screening & Evaluation** Client & Intake worker discuss problem and goals.

Is Treatment Needed? — NO → STOP
YES
Is Optimal Treatment Available At The Center — NO → REFERRAL
YES

2. **Admission to Treatment & Ongoing Evaluation** Decision is made on what services are needed. Case is opened.

3. Which Is Most Appropriate RU? CM* Assigned

4. **Ongoing Treatment, Treatment Plan Formulation & Evaluation** Decisions and ongoing updating of problems, goals, modalities, etc.

5. Is Different Or Additional Assignment Of RU. CM needed? — YES / NO

90-Day Review (In cases where client is in therapy 90 days or more.)

Dropout/ Termination — Are Client's Problems Resolved/ Goals obtained? — NO
YES

6. **CLIENT TERMINATION**

STOP

standardize an operational language for describing problems to be focused on in treatment. Objectives were developed by the clinician with the client and documented on the Direct Service Record (DSR). The problem list, objectives, and LOF were developed as a specific sequential method of describing the assessment results and plan of treatment. The DSR was designed to serve as both an input and output document which records and later displays service data, client data, and financial data for individual clients. It is a duplicate computer form, with the first sheet filed in the client's record as hard copy while the back of the sheet is used for progress notes. The second sheet is used to input client and service data into the computer.

Other forms developed included: (1) The Preliminary Assessment/Program Assignment (PAPA) form which was developed as a tracking mechanism for initial assignment of a client to a treatment program and to a designated case manager following the screening process. Information related to medication, problems, objectives, and initial planned events entered via the PAPA is printed on the DSR form during subsequent services; (2) the Treatment Plan was developed to document and/or modify the significant problems, goals, objectives, and diagnostic information to be focused on in treatment; (3) The Case Management Record was developed as a transfer document after initial program and case manager assignment has occurred; (4) The Discharge Evaluation Record was developed to document a client's formal discharge and closure from the active files of the Center; and (5) The Client Satisfaction Survey was developed as an optional follow-up measure of the level of satisfaction perceived by the client regarding their treatment program. Clinical summary outlines were developed for use at admission, staffing, 90-day review, transfer, and discharge. (See Table 1.)

The automated clinical record system is described in detail in the *Community Health Automated and Record Treatment System (CHARTS) Manual* (Gifford & Maberry, 1979), developed to communicate the sytem to interested groups or agencies. The *CHARTS Training Manual* was written for use in formal training of staff and contains details on completion of forms, appendices of codes, and serves as a staff "users' guide." As components of the system became operational, use of the system was incorporated on a unit by unit basis with training provided at each step of the system's implementation. After approximately one year of development, use, and modifications, center-wide training was provided to all staff using the *CHARTS Manual* and *CHARTS Training Manual*.

Concurrent with the development of the CHARTS System, the financial system was being developed and automated by the Director of Finance together with the software consultants. It is a comprehensive financial system which meets applicable standards of accountability including tracking of expenditure by source of funds linked to identification of specific cost centers called reporting units (RU). In designing the financial accounting system, programs were developed which provided: (1) integrated flexibility in comparing client/ staff service data vs. the cost of providing that service; (2) timely and regular revenue/expenditure reports; and (3) detailed documentation for audit trails.

Along with the development of the demographic, clinical, and fiscal data was the vital requirement that we be able to summarize this data into concise information reports. All levels of staff were involved in designing these reports which helped to ensure their being useful and meaningful to the Center staff, while meeting external reporting requirements.

The process of development, though frustrating and time-consuming, was worthwhile because it provided an opportunity for examining every aspect of the Center's operations for rationale, thus enhancing communication among all levels of staff at all facility locations. Additionally, it required standardization of the data collected. Turnover of the software consultant managers delayed the de-bugging and ongoing modification of the system. There has been a strong temptation to think the system is complete, when in actuality the de-bugging and monitoring of this process must be continued in a very detailed manner. Ongoing monitoring is necessary to assure that input is accurately recorded and entered into the computer. Only by continuous feedback and analysis of output reports can one eliminate errors in the data collecting process, program design, and inconsistent definitions.

Description of Special Features

The automated system in use at the HOTRMHMR has numerous special features that are critical to service delivery and management. One unique feature of the system is the planned event capability, whereby a clinician can be reminded of any service event. This event can be planned for up to a year by simply coding in the date and activity and the computer will print a reminder on that date. This is presently utilized to notify clinicians of case assignments, scheduled treatment appointments, 90-day reviews, and fee reassessment follow-ups. This function is particularly helpful for a busy staff that is engaged in managing large numbers of clients. The planned event is printed on the DSR and distributed to clinicians prior to the appointment, either on a daily basis for central units or weekly for satellite units.

Another unique feature of the DSR is the visual array of current client and staff data, which includes vital problem oriented record information. Specifically, the preprinted display includes current problems, objectives, status of case, treatment modalities for each problem area including medication, initial and current level of functioning, case manager identification, and future service events planned on a single page. Following the service, the clinician records concisely the service provided; time involved, service provider; recipient codes including client or collaterals involved; appointment codes including scheduled, non-scheduled, cancelled, no-show, or emergency situation; client billing information; and any additional planned service events. A blank DSR is available for walk-in and emergency situations. As planned, the DSR: (1) has virtually eliminated input errors because most of the clinical and demographic information is preprinted; (2) simplifies the recording of clinical service data by using only five to seven numbered codes; (3) simplifies keeping client information current; and (4) contains a summary of the client's complete problem oriented record.

The Level of Functioning (LOF) Scale, one for mental health and one for mental retardaton, assesses the global functioning of each client in nine comprehensive areas. LOF scales are completed at intake, every 90 days, at major treatment junctures, and at discharge. This provides a measure of the client's change in independent functioning over time, serves as an instrument to measure treatment effectiveness and cost of improvement or maintenance, and provides a communication tool as to how healthy or dysfunctional a client might be at any given treatment juncture. It also serves as a method to assess an individual's caseload, a unit's caseload, and/or the caseload of the entire center.

Several summary reports are extremely helpful to the direct service provider in managing his clients and his caseload, to the unit director in supervising his unit, to the program director for managing his program, and to center-wide administration in managing the entire center. These summary reports, described below, are provided regularly to appropriate staff.

The Case Management Listing report is available by individual clinician, by unit, and by program, as well as center-wide, and provides each level of staff with a list of clients for whom they are responsible and contains detailed clinical information about each of the clients. This report has been useful in tracking the case management function and in focusing treatment responsibility. For example, when a clinician plans to leave the center there is a current list of clients for whom a disposition must be made prior to his or her leaving. The manager is thus assured that each of the clients has received a proper disposition and that all necessary information has been communicated.

The Staff Event Listing report is a print-out which shows each service activity by clinician and gives the date, type of service, and length of time that service was provided. Service activity is then summarized by the total time each clinician spent in each service unit. The Staff Event Records report summarizes this same detailed data into the total time spent by type of service activity; for example, twenty-two hours in individual therapy, thirty-six hours in group therapy, etc. These two reports are useful to the direct service provider in monitoring where and in what way they spent their time and are helpful to the manager in assessing workload, kind, and amount of service being provided. This information is routinely summarized for individual clinicians and program directors.

The Client Detail report lists services that the individual client has received during any chosen time period. The services are summarized by worker, by type of service, and by the amount of time involved in each type of service. This report is especially useful in determining high-cost clients; examining efficiency of services for gains accomplished in treatment; and evaluating appropriateness of service for particular problems, diagnoses, or other circumstances.

The Client Summary Profile report summarizes demographic information on 40 different profile elements such as race, sex, age, income, educational level, marital status, etc., of any selected unit(s) or program(s). It can also summarize for any single profile element, such as age, for any of the other 39 profile elements. For example a report was needed for a community group on the Center's services to children. The report was requested and easily prepared, providing a profile for all Center clients age 17 and below — to what unit of the Center they were admitted, census tract, sex ratio, race, income of family, and type of problem for which they were admitted. Only the imagination can limit the numerous ways this demographic data can be used for program analysis, service delivery design, and allocation of resources.

The Service Summary by Unit report summarizes by unit the amount of time spent in each type of service, the number of clients served by each type of service, the total numer of hours (both direct and indirect), and the number of service events by type of service. Unit subtotals are then combined into a center-wide summary by total events, hours, and number of clients serviced for that particular period of time.

The financial component of the automated system is a comprehensive financial system with a Users Guide which fully describes the system and instructs workers on its use. The system provides audit trails on all revenues and expenditures and has been extremely helpful in providing detailed data as well as summarized data for all funding source auditors. Internally, the automated financial system provides each unit director, on a regular basis, a detailed analysis of their revenues and expenditures for the current month and year-to-date. The revenue portion of this report provides by source of funds actual and budgeted revenue with a budget variance amount and percentage for the past month and fiscal year-to-date. The total annual budget is also shown with a percentage of year-to-date actual revenues compared to total budget. For expenditures, the report provides a detailed listing of expenses by line item for the current month and year-to-date. Again, variance amounts and percentages are shown by comparisons of actual expenditures vs. budget. These reports allow management staff current and routine information upon which to plan and make decisions.

Cost outcome analysis thus far has been limited. Software programming is currently being completed to integrate the clinical, client, and fiscal elements. Only recently the Texas Department of Mental Health and Mental Retardation (TDMHMR) developed a method of costing which defines a uniform method of determining cost in two ways. The first is by program category (e.g., screening/referral, outpatient, alternate residential, etc.), with unit cost determined by service type appropriate for the category (e.g., outpatient = server hours, inpatient = clients days). The second is by server type for outpatient and screening/referral categories only (e.g., psychiatric service, psychological service, and service by others).

Cost outcome evaluation at HOTRMHMR is presently being done in a variety of ways. For example, the Client Detail report summarizes all of the services that a particular client has received over a given period of time, by type of service and server type. These data, along with the cost of figures by server type and service type, allow calculation of the cost of providing the services to any particular client. That cost can then be compared to any change in their level of functioning. This capability does allow evaluation of clients receiving expensive services for which there might be less expensive services available with similar outcomes. Other examples include using the cost of providing service along with various service summary reports to evaluate: (1) the need for additional groups, (2) use of other more efficient types of service, (3) the use and cost of billable vs. non-billable services such as telephone counseling, and (4) the loss of revenue if services are provided by a clinician that does not qualify for third-party reimbursement.

Advantages and Disadvantages

The advantages of this system have been both obvious and subtle. The formalization of definitions demanded by the automation process has been positive in and of itself. Careful definition of the discrete data elements of the clients' movement through our mental health system has resulted in uniform reporting. Formalization also necessitated the clinician and the client clearly stating and agreeing upon the problems and objectives to be focused on in treatment. This has reduced complaints from staff, clients, and referral agencies concerning clients' confusion about "What am I doing here?" and "What am I working on?"

Unexpected positive results occurred simply because accurate and complete information was available along with an enabling managerial atmosphere. Providing information to staff with clear, agreed-upon goals and expectations has enhanced the performance of direct service providers and managers. The ability to receive a complete Case Management Listing of clients, their past and current level of functioning, and the last date seen, provides the clinician and supervisor an overview that reduces much of the uncertainty characteristic of staff in public mental health agencies. The understanding that work is open for review has reinforced staff to continue performing their best at all times. Summary information on number of clients and level of functioning allows the balance among units to be monitored and adjusted, thus directing staff energy toward the agency goal of providing service rather than allowing internal squabbles to occur over perceived inequities in work demands.

Tracking of service responsibilities by direct care staff and managers has also improved dramatically. As noted earlier, prior to the Staff/Management Information System's development, it was almost impossible effectively to track all clients, especially with rapid client turnover and heavy caseloads. Coincidental with the development of the S/MIS, a statewide mandate for continuity of care was implemented. This concept is essentially a way of tracking clients with the case manager as coordinator. Since this concept had already been incorporated into the automated data system, it was a simple process to implement the continuity of care mandate. With the S/MIS, each new client is assigned a case manager who has the responsibility for either providing direct services and/or assuring that the client receives the services he needs through the Center and/or through other agencies. This tracking process continues even when responsibility for the client is transferred either internally or externally. Simply stated, with the automated clinical record system, it is easy to track and determine "who is doing what to whom, how often, and with what kind of results."

Training of new staff members has been much easier and more complete with the formalized system. Each new staff member is trained on the use of the information system with the *CHARTS Manual*, the *CHARTS Training Manual*, and audio tapes describing the system. Errors are quickly discovered because the structure and monitoring of the system has both manual and computerized feedback mechanisms.

The amount of information made available has increased tremendously. It has required less clerical staff time for routine data collection, thus freeing them for other duties. Also, since the computer can operate 24-hours a day, high overload periods have been staffed in non-traditional work time, such as after-hours and weekends. Cross-training of other support staff including supervisors, typists, and receptionists has increased flexibility in their role utilization.

Client profile information is helpful in providing information and maintaining interagency relationships with community groups, our own board of directors, funding agencies, state offices, and other external groups seeking to review and/or learn the system. Another capability helpful with public information is the computer-generated mailing lists. The computer can print any amount of pregummed mailing labels which are used for mass distribution of the Center's newspaper, brochures, and other printed materials.

Immediate availability of summary reports is a major advantage of the system. The Center's S/MIS now generates all of the summary reports within five to seven working days after the end of the month. Quarterly and annual reports are prepared in an equally timely fashion.

Strategic and long-term financial planning and budgeting has improved dramatically in the last three years with the automated system. Although our Center has experienced the loss of a major staffing grant and the budget has decreased by 20%, it has been possible for the Center to manage this through attrition and fiscal restraint. Short- and long-term planning was made possible because of accurate and dependable current financial information being available on a monthly basis, as well as staff being able to compare current revenue and expenditures with year-to-date projections.

Even though our computerized system has been designed with flexibility in programming and data elements of documents and summary reporting, our experience has emphasized the fact that the modification process is ongoing. This is due to the continuously changing internal needs for information in a mental health system which has multiple funding sources and auditing requirements. There are also continuing revisions in reporting mandates at the local, state, and federal levels requiring changes in program design, format, and input/output documents to maintain compliance.

Several other factors should be considered prior to deciding to automate. The installation and development of an automated system impacts every aspect of an agency's operation. This disturbs the *status quo* and initially meets with the natural resistance associated with any significant change of a system. Also, during the initial phase of development, it was necessary to maintain a parallel manual system. This produced stress, long hours, and, occasionally, short tempers. Added to that was the inevitable delays in programming, breakdowns in hardware, and confusion over which system was being used that day. Although the process tested the resolve and commitment of staff and management initially, the advantages far outweigh the difficulties of implementation.

Future Issues and Summary

The develoment of an automated system is a dynamic, changing process. For example, the Center has current plans to automate personnel functions providing planned events for performance evaluations; job description reviews; and summarized data regarding turnover, attrition, personnel action evaluations; Center workforce analysis; and personnel and applicant profile reports. This information will aid in reviewing all personnel functions and reduce staff time significantly in preparing numerous reports. The Center is also involved in completing its automated client billing system. The component of the S/MIS will provide current accessible information on client fees, third-party billing, and summary analysis for effective management of client fee income.

Additionally, the Center plans to expand information regarding clients who are screened but not admitted. Without case numbers, client demographic information cannot be collected or profiled in summary form except for hours of service. Since this information would be very helpful in evaluating target population needs, the Center is currently investigating modifications necessary to obtain this information.

As noted, cost outcome analysis is being performed; however, to date it is neither a routine process nor prepared in summary report form. The Center is completing the software necessary to integrate the demographic, clinical and fiscal components of the system in order to obtain routine cost outcome evaluations. This will further enhance the capabilities previously noted by allowing regular and routine reviews of high-cost clients, maximum utilization of resources, needed program modification, and evaluation of effectiveness of treatment regimes from a cost standpoint.

The use of the HOTRMHMR S/MIS has become a positive force toward increasing the knowledge about caseloads, client information, and staff service data. Staff comments of ''How will this be useful to me?'' have been replaced by ''Where is my DSR?'' and ''Where is my 90-day reminder DSR?'' Program planning and procedural changes have been smoothly accomplished by utilization of the routine client and service summary reports. Staff have moved from feeling intimidated by the system to viewing the computer as a necessary tool to provide client services. Routine 90-day review summaries and other planned activities are kept current, which positively reinforces task accomplishment.

As budgets tighten up nationwide for mental health services, information regarding selective criteria for services, staff resources, and effective planning becomes more essential. The S/MIS can fully address these areas and is becoming an indispensible tool for clinicians and administrators as we move into the next decade of providing community mental health services. Medium-size systems, such as ours, can buy package systems and are strongly advised to do so with ongoing consultant programming and redesign capabilities for meeting the unique changing needs of their system. With affordable technology such as the mini-computers now available, the price for comprehensive accountability is within the range of even small to mid-size community mental health centers. The automated management system is not a universal remedy for human delivery system problems; however, it has been this Center's experience that manual systems are rapidly becoming obsolete, time consuming, and inefficient. Manual accessory components are still evident in our own S/MIS. Our experience has revealed that no system is fully capable of 100% data accumulation and retrieval. Approximately 75% of our information is now fully automated.

The automated S/MIS has proven to be an effective and efficient mechanism for transmittal of data and information to the state and other external sources, and it has produced a tremendous amount of useful information internally with a very short turn-around time. It has enhanced client treatment, clinical and fiscal accountability, information for management, and has become an indispensable, supportive tool for the quality of care provided by the staff of this community mental health center.

REFERENCES

Community health automated record and treatment system training manual, Unpublished Manual, 1979. (Available from Heart of Texas Region Mental Health Mental Retardation Center, P.O. Box 1277, Waco, Texas 76703.)

Gifford, S., & Maberry, D. An integrated system for computerized patient records. *Hospital and Community Psychiatry*, 1979, *30*, 532–535.

Gifford, S., Shaw, C., & Newkham, J. *Community health automated record and treatment system* (CHARTS), Unpublished manual, 1979. (Available from Heart of Texas Region Mental Health Mental Retardation Center, P.O. Box 1277, Waco, Texas 76703.)

Meldman, M. J., McFarland, G., & Johnson, E. *The problem-oriented psychiatric index and treatment plans.* St. Louis: The C.V. Mosby Company, 1976.

Newman, F. L., Burwell, B. A., & Underhill, W. R. Program analysis using the client oriented cost outcome system. *Journal of Evaluation and Program Planning*, 1978, *1*, 19–30.

Newman, F. L., & Sorensen, J. E. *The program director's guidebook for the design and management of client oriented systems.* Belmont, CA: Lifetime Learning, Wadsworth Publishers, Inc., 1981.

Schoech, D., & Arangio, T. Computers in the human services. *Social Work,* 1979, *24*, 96–101.

9. COMPUTERIZED INFORMATION SYSTEMS: A PRACTICE ORIENTATION

Joan S. Velasquez, PhD
Mary Martin Lynch, PhD

The nationwide thrust for accountability and the rapid technological computer advances of the last decade have come together at a point in time and have fostered a proliferation of computerized information systems throughout the social services field. The experiences of two public human services departments in a midwestern, metropolitan county will be examined as case examples of the development of such systems. These two agencies, community human services and community corrections departments, will be discussed. (The agencies addressed, Ramsey County Community Human Services and Ramsey County Community Corrections, are located in St. Paul, Minnesota.) The development of their systems will be presented with emphasis on the ethical considerations for managers, workers, and clients alike. An effort will be made to look at this new technology in the light of traditional social work values and ethics. The impact of their differing organizational structures and target populations on the design and implementation of their respective systems will be dealt with. The systems will be seen in their developmental stages; one, the corrections system is department wide and newly designed, the other, the mental health system, is an enhancement of a large system, mature in the young world of computers, ten years in operation. Emphasis will be on practice, on the interaction that occurs between agency and client, and on the

Dr. Velasquez is Director of Research & Evaluation, Ramsey County Community Human Services, 160 E. Kellogg Boulevard, Saint Paul, Minnesota 55101. Dr. Lynch is Director of Research, Evaluation and Planning, Ramsey County Community Corrections, Saint Paul, Minnesota.

ways that a computerized information system can impede and/or improve the quality of that interaction.

The demands for accountability, and a belief that information quickly acquired and disseminated can increase social services accountability capability, were key factors in the development of the information systems in both departments under discussion. That computerized systems can generate large, even monumental, volumes of information is a known fact. That this information is always useful for accountability purposes is a topic of frequent debate (Nolan, 1979). This article will present the argument that the computerized information system can and should be useful for accountability purposes to facilitate decision-making. It will be argued that it can be, at best, helpful in those interactions between agency and client that are the *raison d'etre* of the social services enterprise.

A brief description of each agency under consideration and of their respective information systems will precede a discussion of issues of concern to other social service agencies. Each of these agencies operates independently from one another but is responsible to the County Board of Commissioners through a county executive office.

The Community Human Services Department

The Agency

Prior to 1980, distinct Mental Health and Welfare Departments operated within a single county under the direction of a County Board of Commissioners. Because these Departments served many of the same clients (approximately one third of the Mental Health clients also received social services or financial assistance from the Welfare Department), their catchment areas were identical, and they had overlapping administrative responsibilities, the Board resolved, in 1979, to merge them, to create a single Community Human Services Department. Though distinct divisions continue to provide Mental Health, Social Services, and Income Maintenance, administrative functions, such as management analysis, planning, and evaluation address the entire agency.

Also, in 1979, the state legislature passed the Community Social Services Act, delegating social service funding decisions to County Boards, requiring that these Boards develop comprehensive plans for service programs, and mandating that the effectiveness of all programs funded through the Act be evaluated. The Welfare Department, at the time of the merger, operated several computerized information systems, two of which will be addressed here: a client identification system and a social service activity system. The latter produces state-required reports on title XX-funded services. The County Board requested, prior to the merger, that the Mental Health Department develop computerized management information systems capable of producing the type of information available from the Welfare information systems. A project team, comprised of staff from the merging departments and Data Processing staff (Data Processing is a separate County Department, responsible to the County Board), developed the Mental Health Client System in response to this Board mandate, and is beginning development of the Mental Health Activity System at this time.

The Purpose of the Community Human Services Information Systems

The purpose of these systems is two-fold: 1) to provide relevant information for those who make decisions regarding the funding and management of Mental Health services, and 2) to execute routine operations which would otherwise depend on clerical staff. Through extensive interviews with administrators and clinicians, the Project Team defined these system requirements:

1. Count numbers and types of clients served. These counts are required by funders, and provide program managers with information on client volume and target populations reached.
2. Determine how many Mental Health clients receive Income Maintenance and Social Services.
3. Document types and frequency of services provided: document use of staff time.
4. Provide a data base which can be used to evaluate program effectiveness.
5. Provide information required to bill for services. Medicare, Medicaid, insurance companies or clients may be billed.

The Mental Health Information System: An Enhancement

The systems addressed here contain distinct types of data stored in two separate computer files. Data from either file can be interrelated with data which the other file maintains on the same individual, through assignment of a unique client case number in both files. Data Processing staff recommended that Mental Health client data not be maintained in the Welfare Information File for two reasons. First, searching the lengthy Welfare Information File for Mental Health client counts would make computer runs for these clients more costly than necessary. Second, different information is required to serve clients in different divisions of the Department. For example, history of psychiatric hospitalization and outpatient treatment is relevant to Mental Health clinicians in providing service but would not be appropriate to collect for Public Assistance applicants. Financial eligibility determination, on the other hand, require computerization of data which is not pertinent for Mental

Health clients. Separate files enable more efficient collection of dissimilar data. Where Mental Health staff needed information which was already collected for Welfare clients, the same definitions and codes were used, in order to produce compatible counts and reports.

The Project Team determined that a case number, which would follow the client over time, through all divisions of the Department, must be assigned to each individual in order to obtain counts of clients active with more than one program. The Welfare Department had maintained, for several years, a centralized case clearing/number assignment function, based on careful identification of each new application and a subsequent search of the entire file for previous contact with the Department. Individuals who appeared on the file retained their original case numbers; new numbers were assigned to new applicants. Mental Health clients now receive case numbers through the same process. Though data regarding these clients is entered in a separate file, their numbers appear on the Welfare Information System, accompanied by a confidential code which blocks access to their data by anyone, other than Mental Health & Information System staff.

The Mental Health Client System includes demographic, client characteristic, and background information provided through client-completed forms obtained prior to the Intake interview. The Mental Health Activity System will report information related to client services: who was seen, by whom, for what length of time, what service was provided, at what cost. Cost figures are obtained by aggregating time spent by professional staff in providing services, then dividing by funds allocated to that service program.

By interrelating data in both Mental Health files, decision-makers may receive reports regarding types of services provided to specific individuals, or types of individuals (elderly, minorities, the severely mentally ill, for example), reports distributing staff time across a variety of services, or cost of providing selected services to various target populations.

The Community Corrections Department

The Agency

The Community Corrections Department under consideration has evolved through a series of departmental reorganizations and mergers into a countywide agency, which provides, detention, probation, and parole services for juvenile and adult offenders, as well as domestic relations services for parents and children involved with the family court. The department has several widely dispersed sites of operation which are relatively dissimilar and autonomous in relation to one another. The department is funded from county (70%) and state resources (30%). It responds, through the County Executive Director's Office, to the County Commissioners and to the State, through the

State Department of Corrections, which is mandated to manage the County's relationship to requirements of the Community Corrections Act. It also has a primary responsibliity to serve the Municipal and the District Courts. Although the Courts have no fiscal relationship with the Department, they do have appointing authority to departmental administrators and are heavily involved in the Justice Advisory Board, which oversees the Department's involvement regarding the Community Corrections Act subsidy which, as noted above, accounts for nearly a third of the departmental budget.

The Community Corrections Department responds to information requests from the State Correctional Department and the Bureau of Criminal Apprehension. It has a mandate from State and County government to develop a management information system. After several abortive attempts to develop such a system, the department contracted with a management systems consulting firm to work with the department in the design, development, and implementation of the Community Corrections Information System (hereafter, referred to as the CCIS). The design and development have been completed and implementation is in process. The Research and Evaluation Unit of the Corrections Department, staff of the County Data Processing Department, and staff of the consulting firm have worked as a team in the development and implementation of this system.

The Purposes of the Community Corrections Information System

The Community Corrections Information System (CCIS) was designed to enable Community Corrections Department staff to track the process of a client through its system for the purposes of providing information for:

1. On-line workers
2. Planners, managers, and administrators
3. Evaluation and Research staff
4. Advisory and County Board decision-makers
5. State and Federal agencies with reporting requirements

The Community Corrections Information System: A New Development

The CCIS, like the Mental Health Client System, contains separate computer files holding different types of data. These files contain client, services, and staff data, as well as client event and client history data. The data in the master files, the maintenance of these files, and the reporting of ongoing events are provided by each decentralized unit to a central control unit. This central control unit assembles input for daily submissions to the Data Processing Department. Following the computer process, daily, weekly, and other periodic reports are generated and distributed through the control unit.

The CCIS establishes and maintains a constant case number for each client to provide for the possibilities of identifying clients by family and of cross-referencing to other systems which use case numbers. The system uses a general purpose report generator to meet ad hoc, infrequent requests for statistical reports. The CCIS has been developed to allow for expansion in the areas of evaluation information collection and processing, on-line access, and interface with other criminal justice information systems.

Technology in Service to Practice

Computerized information systems in the public social services sector serve as a tool in the management and delivery of services. It is essential that this "tool" not be viewed as a neutral instrument to be tolerated or ignored. Such systems call for analysis—from the same ethical and value base as other social work interventions; they should be scrutinized with as much care as that which is given to the interactions between workers and clients. The following discussions around the issues of organizational environment, program evaluation, confidentiality, and barriers to service will be presented from the perspective of the social work practitioner. The reader is asked to recall professional commitments to self-determination, privacy, and social justice and apply them to these case examples of information system development.

Organizational Environment and Structure

The two agencies under consideration serve specialized populations in a decentralized organizational structure.

Community Human Services: Mental Health

The Mental Health Clinic directs services primarily toward low to moderate income individuals and families who are experiencing acute symptoms or crises. Most services are provided at the Clinic, although several specialized programs are housed at other locations. Because clients may be active with several programs at the same time, managers need to know which programs provide what services, for which clients, in order to ensure coordination. Thus, a service recording system is essential.

Incorporating five decentralized programs operated by the Clinic into one information system raised numerous procedural problems. Clinic procedures were developed to collect data from individuals who come to this location for service, whereas two of the de-centralized programs have a strong outreach component, with most client contact occurring outside the office. Consequently, Clinic procedures could not apply to these programs. The organizational structure called for development of different procedures for each decentralized program. A technical perspective tempts project staff to standardize the system for all programs, often changing service delivery in the process. The Team for this project took a strong stand against altering service processes to accommodate data collection. The result is a somewhat more complex and costly system. One decentralized program provides extensive crisis telephone counseling, plus community education. This program was excluded from the computerized information system, since obtaining the required data would intrude unnecessarily into clients' lives and interfere with service. Program staff maintain manual client counts.

Community Corrections Department

The organizational structure of an agency will influence which type of system is selected to meet informational needs in the design phase of the project. The primary options available are a batch, or an on-line system. In a batch system, information is written on paper forms, gathered into "batches" of forms, keypunched into computer-readiness form, processed by the computer, compiled for printing into paper reports or for retrieval by terminal and, finally, stored for aggregation and future retrieval. In an on-line system, information is typed into the terminal, processed by the computer and stored for retrieval by users, by means of typing in requests which can be answered on the terminal or printed out in paper reports if desired. The information will also be stored for aggregation and future retrieval.

The batch system is typical of some of the earlier computerized information systems, which were developed in the mid to late seventies. The system relied on a single and costly computer in a centralized data processing agency. Terminals which could relay information directly to the computer and relay the resultant reports back through the terminals have been prohibitively expensive until the last year. The cost of the personal effort in compiling, punching, and transporting was far less than the cost of computing. Thus, large complicated systems, such as those developed by both agencies under discussion, were dependent on heavy effort in batching, and punching information and transporting reports. The Welfare Department System, on which the Mental Health Client System is based, used a batch process, but also used on-line terminals to access much of the information that was especially pertinent to line staff.

The on-line system is typical of more recent or, earlier, but more costly, systems. Such a system relies on access to terminals to input information and to access the desired information following computer processing. The cost of computing has decreased in recent years (due to improved technology), while the relative cost of personnel has increased.

The need for varying degress of interaction between divisions in the Corrections Department, which are geographically decentralized, indicate a structure which would lend itself to a totally "on-line" system. Each site would input information regarding client activity on a continuous basis and would access report data, as needed. For example, when a recently convicted offender is brought to the County Detention facility from the Court, the decisions as to living arrangement, case work treatment, work, and education planning, which have to be made very quickly, would be greatly facilitated by an immediate ability to access an updated report of a client's past history and current investigation. Such a capability is available with an "on-line" system. At the point in time that this system was being designed, the cost of terminals for the many sites which must input data was prohibitively costly. Consequently, a batch system was chosen, not for functional reasons, but due to cost constraints. The scope of the project was such that by the time the system was to be implemented, more than two years had elapsed and the cost of an on-line system had decreased enough to have made such a system feasible. The anticipated delay and confusion of such a major design shift led the department to accept the consulting firm's advice to continue with the batch system, as originally designed.

It is difficult to assess the correctness of this decision; however, it is possible to look at this experience for lessons regarding future MIS-decisions. Technological advance has been rapid in computer systems; and there is no evidence that such advances are on the wane. County governments should understand this basic fact as they make Data Processing decisions. Development or modification projects should be defined in discreet segments that do not require long term efforts that are more than 6 to 12 months—efforts which may quickly become unnecessary in the face of another technological improvement in computer capability. Thus, the two-year investment in the CCIS, in terms of dollars and education and involvement of users would not outweigh the clear advantages of a decentralized, on-line system, which is now more financially accessible. Recent analysis of computer use (Schoech & Schkade, 1980) indicates that the confidence of users in the system is the key factor in data reliability and consequently validity. To expect high involvement of users in the implementation of a system they already know is out of date is not realistic. The workers in the Corrections Department are familiar with highly automated systems in the commercial world and expect comparable capability in a system which they see consuming great energy and money within the agency. The confidence necessary to ensure reliable input that will produce reliable reports require a staff that believes that the system is "worthwhile."

Program Evaluation

Legislative mandates to evaluate effectiveness of social service programs, plus a commitment to program evaluation on the part of the County Board, provided an impetus for both departments under discussion to develop information systems which provide a data base for evaluation. There is also a concern within each department that evaluation efforts are not only a reflexive reaction to external pressure, but that there is genuine input from and feedback to practitioners.

It is in such a spirit that both departments are implementing a formative approach to program evaluation. Based on the premise that program improvement is a primary purpose for evaluation, a formative approach involves ongoing data collection and periodic feedback to staff regarding program performance. Evaluators assist program staff to delineate their services and target populations, clarify program goals and objectives, and establish a data collection system. Data regarding the extent to which objectives are accomplished is summarized on a quarterly basis and reviewed by staff and others who make decisions regarding that program. Evaluations focus primarily on client outcome objectives. Improved functioning, obtaining employment, or movement to a less supervised setting are typical mental health client outcomes. These, plus recidivism, are used for correctional evaluations. The formative evaluation is designed to serve three functions:

1. Accountability: funders, consumers, service providers want to know what programs accomplish.

2. Improve program performance: program staff use data to determine what changes are necessary, if programs do not perform as well as expected. Worker self assessment is encouraged.

3. Planning: policy makers assess a program's compatibility with over-all service goals to consider necessary modification and changes in the service system.

Mental Health Outcome Data

The Mental Health Information systems are able to support basic formative evaluation which focuses on effort or outcome.

For example, programs may set objectives regarding which target populations to reach, how many clients to serve, or which services should consume staff time. Together, the client and activity systems provide the data base for measuring these effort-related objectives.

To measure client outcome for Mental Health Services, a set of Level of Functioning Scales is being developed for each target population served by the Department (Velasquez, 1979). Clinicians rate client functioning at Intake, on a set of dimensions such as social interaction, personal care, decision-making, employment. This initial rating becomes a part of the Mental Health Client System and is used to describe the client population in terms of current functioning. The project staff is developing procedures for periodic recording of these scales at case review and termination, in order to use them as a measure of client change.

Additional client outcome data, such as reduction of violence in Abuse cases, can be added to the sub-file as evaluation is expanded. All outcome data can be interrelated with client characteristic or activity information in response to questions regarding amount of effort required to achieve specified outcomes for various client populations.

Community Corrections Outcome Measure Development

The CCIS contains basic client services and work data that are useful measures of program effort. Data relating to recidivism, the most common outcome measure in criminal justice evaluation and research, is available in great detail and refinement. Recidivism, typically defined as subsequent convictions with a time-limiting factor, has shortcomings as an outcome measure of program success. An undue emphasis on such a measure may well ignore intervening forces and imply a cause and effect relationship that may well not exist. Therefore, the system is designed in such a way that the services items currently collected can be assigned outcome codes such as those existing in the Mental Health Client System. This type of individualized and refined outcome measurement should yield more programmatically useful data. Such an enhancement is foreseen in the systems modification phase of the development of the CCIS.

Considerable assessment work has been underway throughout the divisions. Both the juvenile and adult residential institutions have carefully developed a classificaton and level of functioning system which is used in placement, treatment and case planning. The juvenile residential facility uses the Jesness outcome measures to assess client development (Jesness, 1972). The assessment of behavior determines the type of living arrangement and treatment a juvenile experiences in the facility. The treatment work there and in the adult facility reflects years of developmental work which incorporates the pre-treatment and post-treatment testing of clients. The juvenile facility uses the Jesness Inventory to assess delinquency tendencies. Other divisions have also adopted and/or modified other treatment theories into their probationary and diversion work. The true test of the CCIS's usefulness, in regard to evaluation, will be in its capability to incorporate and build on this practice-based assessment capability. The workers and psychologists in these programs are sophisticated researcher/practitioners. They have used their skill to treat clients and to assess the impact of that treatment on these individuals. The burden rests with those managing the information system to use these tools to broaden the assessment of individual clients to the assessment of programs. The information system can be used to minimize the data collection process, to allow for speedy aggregation and statistical analysis, and to generate timely and reliable reports; the CCIS, and any computerized system, can accomplish such technical feats, but the information system designers must watch for the practice skill in individual client assessment and incorporate such information into a system to ensure that it can be aggregated for program evaluation. Workers have traditionally resisted the type of outcome measures that too frequently are imposed on them as indications of the effectiveness of their programs. The achievement/non-achievement dichotomous measures associated with Title XX evaluation requirements have disenchanted workers who deal in a far richer and more complex reality.

It is unethical to measure program performance superficially. It is unethical to collect and aggregate program performance information that doesn't reflect the complexities of practice. These programs impact deeply on the life experience of clients. To discontinue, modify *or* continue any service casually is a disservice to client and taxpayer alike. The CCIS, as well as other computerized information systems, must be designed to reflect and enhance the sophistication of practice assessment. Practitioners in both Departments have expressed a willingness to cooperate in the development of the information and formative evaluation systems. They become enthusiastic regarding the potential for feedback and self-correction, when they sense these systems can reflect the nuances of their practice. It is at such a point that program evaluation begins to serve clients and workers as well as management decision-makers.

Confidentiality

Concern regarding the rights of individuals to control information about themselves has resulted in extensive privacy legislation at all levels of government. The state's data privacy law has moved all government agencies to critique their behavior regarding the privacy rights of their clients. The Community Corrections and Community Human Services Departments are no exception in this regard. Each deparment shares some of the common problems of confidentiality that have long been of concern to the social work profession. The tension between organizational pressure for accountability and cost effectiveness and professional desire for highly personalized and voluntary interactions are shared by the two departments. However, each department also has problems unique to the characteristics of their target population.

Community Corrections Department: A Captive Client

The Corrections client enters the department because of an action of the Court, or in anticipation of such an action in the case of diversion and domestic relations services. The client is captive; his or her involvement is typically mandated by the Court and a lack of what is defined as ''appropriate'' involvement can result in more severe action from the Court. The punishment function of Corrections work is a strong one, as is the function of rehabilitation and removal from society. The tendency has frequently been to forget that the privacy and confidentiality rights of clients, while not as clear as for other social services clients, still exist and must be honored. In fact, the vulnerability of the Correctional clients to inappropriate use of recorded information is undoubtedly greater. An offender's ''record'' is frequently the basis for judgments regarding the severity and length of sentence. The accuracy of that record is of great significance. The right of offenders to access their records, to question their accuracy, and to demand the correction of errors is one to be protected conscientiously.

Elaborate procedures have been developed to ensure that the clients with information about them in the CCIS have these rights. Workers who are expected to provide detailed pre-sentence investigation to the Courts and to be aware of the details of the lives of their probationers and parolees may well find these procedures cumbersome, or even counter-productive. The CCIS managers are responsible for streamlining these procedures and for assisting staff to appreciate the necessity of such procedures. The Correctional worker has to be supported in dealing with their sometimes conflicting responsibilities to the Courts, the clients, and to society as a whole.

The issues of confidentiality are especially complex in regard to juveniles who enter the Correctional system. A historic confusion as to the status of such juveniles exists. The conflict as to whether these young people should be dealt with as criminals in need of removal from society and of punishment, or as clients in need of rehabilitation, has never been definitively resolved. It is argued that their status as client has resulted in treatment that does not provide them with due process. It has also been argued that their status as client has resulted in shielding some juveniles from the just penalties for crimes committed. The design of the CCIS has forced decisions around juvenile records that have highlighted these conflicts. A master index of client data had been designed to incorporate all individuals served by the department, adults and juveniles alike. This index contains detailed demographic and service data and was to be accessible to all workers. Privacy concerns were raised, the agency's privacy and security group convened, and the issue was resolved. The juvenile judge and Corrections staff were forced to plunge into the issue of privacy of juveniles and to decide how that privacy can be best protected. Juvenile records have been separated from adults on the index and access to them has been carefully controlled.

Many juveniles enter and leave the system without ever being adjudicated. The treatment of records regarding such juveniles also became a concern of the CCIS managers. The past record of current offenders is of intense interest to judges in the Courts. Recent state law has set down guidelines regarding the weighting of past offenses in assigning sentences for particular crimes. The role of the records of non-adjudicated youth, in relation to pre-sentence investigations, became another serious policy decision for the Courts and the Department. The development of the CCIS forced consideration of the issue.

Purging and sealing decisions had to be made. The concern for the rights of the youth and the need of the Department to be responsive to the requests of the Courts informed the decision. The commitment of social work practitioners to ensure the privacy of the client whenever possible was instrumental in the decision to destroy all records of non-adjudicated youth upon their eighteenth birthday. The legal situation, the onset of CCIS implementation, and the willingness of staff to assess the situation from a values perspective came together to effect a coherent policy regarding access to juvenile records.

Mental Health Clients: The Right to Privacy

Because all Mental Health client information is considered confidential, both the fact that an individual receives Mental Health services and data regarding that individual are protected. The Project Team attempted to balance the need for data with the client's right to privacy. Since many Mental Health clients are County employees, clinical staff were particularly concerned that client status not be available to other employees. This information is protected by adding a confidential code to numbers assigned through Mental Health. Only Clinic staff and a minimal number of information system staff can access the names or other data attached to these case numbers. When clients complete Intake documents, the secretary asks them to read and sign a statement indicating who may have access to the information they provide.

Barriers to Service: A Mental Health Dilemma

Ensuring that computerized information systems not create barriers to service is primarily a Mental Health, rather than a Corrections issue. The intent of Mental Health programs is to provide services which alleviate crises and maintain or increase the client's capacity to function. The information system is intended to aid in the management of these programs with minimal intrusion into the process of service delivery.

The Project Team attempted to balance the need for consistent data collection, with the requirement that the information system not interfere with services. As a result of extensive interviews with clinicians and lengthy observation of the flow of clients and their data through the Clinic, the Team made these decisions: 1) Develop one set of information system input documents to collect client data at one point in time. These forms (completed in triplicate) serve as the Intake facesheet for the client's record, provide background information for the Clinician, include data necessary for accurate case number assignment, and meet the billing department's requirements. 2) Simplify these documents and request that the client complete them while waiting to be interviewed. The Secretary greets the client, requests completion of two forms, and offers to answer any questions. Costly staff time is saved by asking clients to complete forms, and client privacy is protected. 3) Do not collect data items unless their use can be justified. After requesting that managers and clinical staff identify their information needs, Project Team members asked that they consider how an aggregate count of that item would be useful in managing programs. Several "interesting to know" items were discarded. Including Clinical staff in these decisions and approaching the system from the perspective of usefulness diminished inherent resistance to developing a computerized system. 4) Consistently consult with clerical staff who will be responsible for obtaining and maintaining correct data and distributing it. These staff members have daily involvement with the information system. Incorporating their suggestions not only results in more sensible procedures, but increases their sense of control over assigned tasks.

Though the Mental Health and Welfare systems have common general purposes, specific information needs and constraints vary, due to differences across programs in target populations and types of services provided. These variations were accommodated through construction of separate, but compatible data files, designed to produce similar management reports. However, one aspect of standardization, the process for assigning case numbers, proved to be unavoidable and has created a major problem. Several specific data items are required by the Welfare Clearing System, in order to assign a unique case number. This system was designed to prevent fraud through collection of duplicate payments and is highly accurate. Whereas Public Assistance may be legitimately withheld where information is not provided, insistence on such requests creates an unacceptable barrier to accessible Mental Health services. Nearly 10% of the Mental Health clients refuse or cannot respond to two data items required to clear a case on the Welfare Information System: name of divorced spouse and birthdates of parents. Although these data have no relevance to clinical services, they are required for case number assignment. Rather than create a barrier to service for these clients, by insisting on responses to these items, a manual system is currently operated to count and bill for them. However, maintenance of this manual system, in addition to the computerized system, increases the support staff workload, and diminishes the accuracy of billing and evaluative information. Project staff are experimenting with alternative procedures, which will allow entry of incomplete data onto the file and, thus, incorporate 100% of the clients into the computerized system.

The dilemma encountered in attempting to integrate systems whose original purposes are divergent must be carefully addressed whenever merging of Departments or functions is considered.

Credibility of data on which service-oriented decisions will be based must also be addressed. Since Managers intend to use the information systems as a data base for decision-making, the data must be as complete and accurate as possible. The Project Team began with the premise that data would be incomplete if procedures were complex or incompatible with service practices, or if staff responsible for supporting input did not find the system useful. To expect, at the onset, that a service oriented staff will enthusiastically embrace a computerized information system is naive and unrealistic. However, if the system substitutes for work completed manually, or produces useful reports, our experience indicates that staff will conscientiously support an accurate data base. Involving Direct Service and Clerical staff throughout the Project increases the likelihood that the system will meet their needs, will be based on sensible procedures, and consequently, produce more credible data.

Summary

At a time when accountability and evaluation are mandated and funding is austere, human service agencies are looking toward computerized information systems for establishing accountability and for assistance in decision-making. The extensive, complex data which can be stored and retrieved through a computerized system can provide an invaluable information base for agency management. A social service practice orientation demands that those who develop and implement these systems consider the ethics and values which guide interaction between agency and client, to create an emphasis on enhancing rather than impeding the quality of service provided.

REFERENCES

Jesness, C. F., DeRisi, W., McCormick, P., & Wedge, R. *The youth center project: Final report*. Sacramento: California Youth Authority and American Justice Institute, 1972.

Nolan, R. L. Managing the crises in data processing. *Harvard Business Review*, 1979, *57*, 115–126.

Schoech, D. J., & Schkade, L. L. What human services can learn from business about computerization. *Public Welfare*, 1980, *38*, 18–27.

Velasquez, J. S. *An experimental evaluation of milieu therapy in a community-based residence*. Unpublished doctoral dissertation, University of Minnesota, 1979.

10. AN INFORMATION SYSTEM
FOR THE SOCIAL CASEWORK AGENCY:
A MODEL AND CASE STUDY

Bruce A. Phillips, PhD
Bernard Dimsdale, PhD
Ethel Taft, MSW

In the fall of 1976, the Planning Department of the Jewish Federation-Council of Greater Los Angeles charged its research specialist with developing some means of collecting service delivery data that would be accurate, flexible, and produce reports within time limits imposed by the decision-making process. As a result of preliminary exploration with the casework agencies funded by JFC, it was clear that these agencies were acutely aware of the shortcomings of their current manual systems; both in terms of providing planning data and in terms of providing internal management data.

All four major casework agencies (Jewish Family Service of Los Angeles, Jewish Family Service of Santa Monica, Jewish Big Brothers, and Jewish Vocational Service) agreed to develop a unified system which would encompass the needs of all of them. The Research Specialist began by working independently with each of the four agencies to begin to map out a common ground. After several months, it appeared that a unified information structure would be feasible and workable for the four casework agencies. A demonstration grant was secured to develop the system at this point. A systems designer was brought in to work together with the research specialist in coordinating the further development of a unified system.

In this paper, we will describe the development of the Jewish Family Service of Los Angeles component because the work characterizes the process as a whole.

Dr. Phillips is Assistant Professor, Hebrew Union College-Jewish Institute of Religion, 3077 University Ave., Los Angeles, CA 90007. Dr. Dimsdale is a consultant in Applied Mathematics and Data Processing. Ms. Taft is Assistant Director for the Jewish Family Service of Los Angeles.

Identifying Information Requirements

The first step in designing an information system is to determine the information needed. This was accomplished by setting up an interdisciplinary task-group, made up of three components: the research specialist, the systems designer, and agency personnel. Their functions were as follows:

Research Specialist

1. Represented the information of the Planning and Budgeting Department.
2. Provided expertise on problems of data collection.
3. Coordinated JFS component with other agencies within the system.

Agency Director, Associate and Assistant Directors

1. Interpreted information required of agency by United Way.
2. Interpreted information most useful for setting and implementing agency policy.
3. Determining information usable for agency planning.

Agency District Directors

1. Interpreted information useful for worker, supervisor and district administration.
2. Provided expertise on data collection problems and procedures within District Office.

Systems Designer

1. Translated information requirements into data processing considerations.
2. Provided feedback to task group on feasibility and cost of suggestions made.
3. Design of system when requirements finalized.
4. Supervised programming and testing of final system.

The process of defining the system, then, involved exploration, feedback, synthesis, and negotiation. As the two technical personnel learned more about the agency (agencies), the agency personnel were sensitized to technical considerations. As a result, the technical personnel suggested new system applications based on a greater understanding of the agency, and the agency personnel focused more clearly on the relative signficance of various requests as they became more familiar with system capabilities.

In addition, input was included from line workers, clerical staff as well as members of lay committees in the Planning and Budgeting Departments and the agency (agencies).

In order to promote creativity and an optimally useful system, task force participants were encouraged to "think big." When the lists of information required were laid on the table, it was clear that there was far more than could be included. In order to separate essential information from "would be nice to have," three criteria were developed.

1. *Usability:* How would the proposed information be used, and what sorts of decisions might be made on the basis of this information. There was strong feeling, for example, that certain kinds of clinical data should be included in the system. For example, information, about significant others in the client's immediate constellation of friends and relatives. On closer inspection, however, it became clear that this information would not be used for any application other than the worker's own edification. Instead, a new form was added to the case folder, summarizing this information for the worker's use.

2. *Appropriateness to Computerization:* Could this information be handled as well without being part of a computerized system? The telephone receptionist, for example, records requests for information by putting "hash marks" on a piece of paper. Since it was determined that no further detail was required (such as the kinds of information requested, the referral made by the receptionist, or the time taken in making the referral), it was deemed more appropriate to keep this process separate from the computer systems.

3. *Computer System Implications:* The most important of which is cost. Is the cost of collection and storage warranted by the usability of the information? Does inclusion of this data present any data collection or computer systems problems? The task group decided that five generic types of information met these criteria, and were essential for inclusion in the system:

  (a) *Caseflow:* Data such as the number of open cases, number of new cases, number of closed cases, number of active cases, and other monthly activity information.

  (b) *Case Profile:* For example, composition of the family being served, focus of service, family income, etc.

  (c) *Relation of Case to Larger Social Welfare System:* Here we were interested in tie-ins between the agency and the larger social service network. Included here is information relevant to source of referral, destination of referral out, other welfare services received (AFDC, SSI, etc.).

  (d) *Cumulative data about service modalities* used over the life of the case.

  (e) *The cost of direct service,* as measured by casework time spent on the case.

The discussion process described above can continue indefinitely. For this reason, the technical personnel established two criteria for determining finalization.

First, there was no longer any empirical way of resolving uncertainties. The only questions left were speculations about what might happen, or what might turn out to be the best information to have collected. This would become apparent only after a system was in operation for some time.

Second, there was already sufficient consensus achieved within the task group about the general structure of the system, so that individual differences appear to be minimal.

The source of referral codes are a good case in point. Much discussion had taken place over appropriate codes for source of referral. Some members felt there were too many, others felt the list to be incomplete. Still others disagreed with the whole classification schema. Because this issue did not affect the overall structure of the system, it was decided to use the codes as they had been developed so far and then see which ones actually were used, and what new ones might be needed.

The focus of services codes also illustrates the role of the systems designer. If up to 9 codes are used, the computer stores one digit, if between 10 and 99 codes are used, two digits are required. The systems designer pointed out that an exact set of codes was not important for systems purposes and new codes could be added later.

Once the system is finalized, the basic logic of the system cannot be changed without substantial expense. in the example of changing codes cited above, the basic logic of the system was unaffected. Adding essentially different information can alter the basic logic: for example, after programming had begun, some task group members decided to add a new piece of information requiring only one additional digit on the intake form. The systems designer pointed out that making this change would involve significant reprogramming, resulting in a substantial increase in programming cost (not to mention printing new forms). The impulse to redesign the system after it was underway created confusion, uncertainty, and almost negated the lengthy process that had gone before. Only the systems designer has the technical expertise to judge between a trivial change and a major one. Rather than debating the merits of this proposed change, the task group should have first consulted the systems designer about its practicability. As a result of this misadventure, it was decided to create a monitoring committee to review the system and propose changes for eventual production of a modified system based on actual experience with the present system.

In this first section we have used our own experience to develop a model for deciding on informational requirements. In the next section, we describe the administrative structure of the system along with the kinds of decisions that were made in determining it.

The Administrative Structure of the System

The flow of information is based on the case cycle itself. Thus, when a case is opened, an intake document is filled out. The actual casework activity is recorded on contact slips. The case is closed by submitting a closing document, and can be reopened again with a new intake. In addition, there is an intake change form which can modify the contents of the intake sheet in the master file. (See the next section for more about the master file). When a case is transferred to a new worker, for example, an intake change form would be used. In the following discussion, both the function and content of each type of document will be discussed along with the most pertinent decisions.

Intake Form

The intake form opens a case for the computer and also serves as a face sheet on the case. By combining the face sheet with the input document, we were able to avoid adding yet another piece of paper for the clerical staff to handle as part of the intake process. The workers had long desired some organized way of recording additional information about the client which was pertinent only to clinical aspects of the case. As a result of designing the computer intake form, a second form providing this background information was added to the intake process for inclusion in the case folder only. Thus, a long felt clinical need was addressed as a result of developing the computerized system.

In considering the actual content of the intake form, the task group found it necessary to make a disinction between a "case" and a "client." In the past, the agency itself had never been consistent in how it classified family members. In some instances, the entire family constituted the case, while in other instances each individual family member was considered to be a case (and given an individual case identifying number). Giving careful consideration both to how the data would be used and the implications for the system design, it was decided that the family should be the case, because the family is the specified unit of service for the agency. The systems designer translated this distinction into computer terms and made it possible to record information about the individual family members within the case. Thus, the system can count cases, clients, as well as other family members not seen as clients.

The task group then had to decide what information to collect about the case and what information to collect about family members.

Two constraints set limits on the amount of information to be included. First, it was desirable to minimize worker time involved in filling out the intake form. Each additional item on the intake increases worker resistance, collection costs (in worker time), and processing costs (in computer time). Second, it was felt that an increase in information would result in a decrease in accuracy. The task force agreed to include the following information components on the intake sheet (in order of their appearance on the form):

—Agency
—Form type (Intake)
—District within agency
—Case ID
—ID check (first three letters of principal client surname)
—Worker ID (worker to whom case is assigned)
—Date of transaction (i.e., date of request for service)
—Date of last close (if this is a reopened case)
—Source of referral
—Family income
—Zip code of residence
—Applicable insurance carried
—Tie-ins with public welfare system (such SSI, AFDC, Medicare, etc.)
—Primary focus of service
—Secondary focus of service
—Number of children in the household ages 13–18
—Number of children in the household under 13
—Number of children in the household who are seen as clients
—Sex, marital status, client status, and date of birth for each adult in household

In order to reduce the amount of effort involved in filling out the forms, the first three items (Agency, Form Type and District) are pre-printed. Each worker is provided with an ID stamp and a date stamp. This is true for all the forms used in the system. A Rolodex is provided to each worker for looking up client ID's.

Two of these items required much discussion before a decision could be made. These are reviewed here in some detail because they illustrate the kinds of conceptual problems that are raised in the process of developing an information system. The focus of service for a case had traditionally been noted on the face sheet using standard FSAA codes. The possibilities inherent in a computerized system triggered a re-evaluation both of the standard codes and of the very process of defining focus of service. Because the focus of service can change over the life of an episode, the task group wished to have this case dynamic reflected in the system. Rather than record the focus of service at intake, the JFS participants in the task group wanted to record the focus of service for each contact. Then, the question was raised: "Why just one focus of service per contact, when, after all, two or three issues might be raised in the course of a session?" As the research specialist and systems designer pointed out, the worker time involved to record all this plus the additional storage costs made this approach unfeasible. Finally, even if these considerations were not obstacles, the likelihood that no single focus of service would ever develop from all this detail further argued against this approach.

Instead the technical members suggested that greater confidence be placed in the clinical judgment of the worker in determining focus of service which could be included in the system by adding a retrospective assessment of the focus of service made at the time of closing. It was also decided to stick with the basic FSAA codes and to augment them with special codes reflecting services unique to the agency (for the most part, these are concrete services provided by the agency such as conservatorship, locating board and care homes and the like).

Intake Change Form

The intake change form is used to change information originally submitted on the intake form. It is identical in appearance with the intake form with three exceptions. Document type indicates intake change (necessary for data processing), date of change replaces data of request for service, and new ID check replaces date of last closing.

Contact Slip

The largest single obstacle to implementation of the system was finding a way to collect data about case activity. Two of the central purposes of the system discussed above were to record the modalities used and the amount of time spent in direct service. The only way to accomplish this is to collect information about activity at the time it takes place. The most efficient method was immediately determined to be a contact slip filled out for each contact. The workers, however, resisted this idea, and a number of alternative methods were then explored, and tested, and rejected. Every other method ended up taking more time and being less economical than the contact slip (especially with pre-pointed fields and data stamps). The objection was less to the contact slip itself, than to the change it represented from the way the manual system operated (using a monthly summary sheet). Suddenly, the manual system which was generally agreed to be awkward, inaccurate, and inefficient seemed attractive. Ultimately, the executive staff of the agency had to decide that this would be the way to go. Interestingly, the contact slips have not been a problem; rather the major problem with the system is that the workers fill out contact slips for cases which they have neglected to open in the first place.

The contact slip, like the intake document, includes agency, form type, district, case ID, ID check, worker ID, and date of transaction (date of contact).

There are seven codes for type of contact listed on the contact slip: individual, joint (i.e., couple), family, home visit, group, significant telephone, and "other." The inclusion of "significant telephone" and "other" added two types of contact not included in the manual system. "Significant telephone'' is used for direct service that takes place over the phone (as opposed to making appointments). ''Other'' is used for collateral activity on behalf of the case. While not direct in the strictest clinical sense of the term, this category allows for inclusion of all other activity related to the case, which results in direct service being provided to the client(s). The type of contact is coded as a single letter and entered this way on the slip. The time spent on the contact is recorded in hours and minutes. The contact slip also includes agency, form type (contact), district, client ID, ID check, worker ID, and date of transaction (contact).

Closing Form

The closing form summarizes information about the conclusion of the case. As with the other two forms, the closing document begins with agency, form type (closing), district case ID, ID check, worker ID, and date of transaction (date of closing). The closing document also records:

—who closed the case (worker, client, or both)
—reason for closing
—referral out (if closed by referral)
—basis and type of financial aid given (if any)
—fee information
—workers closing assssment of principal focus of service

The development of codes for reasons for closing, like the focus of service codes, triggered the agency to re-evaluate the implications of the traditional closing codes used. The first step in this process was a differentiation between clinical and concrete services. Concrete services are essentially closed by one code: ''service completed,'' to indicate that the needed help was rendered. The clinical codes posed more of a problem. The old code ''problem resolved'' was recognized to be inappropriate for a short term agency (in addition to the clinical problem of this determination). ''Situation improved'' was substituted instead. In addition, to describe more realistically the reason for closing, the following codes were added: ''client not satisfied with service,'' ''service no longer desired/situation changed,'' ''person(s) assessed as not treatable,'' ''no resource in community/client refuses service.''

These codes were worded so as to provide as much detail as possible without seeming to evaluate the worker. Evaluation is a separate process from management information. Moreover, if the closing document seemed to be evaluating the worker, all cases would end up being closed with ''problem resolved.''

In addition to clinical reasons for closing a case, it was realized that there also exist reasons for closing that are external to the case, and which have important implications for agency planning. These are "client cannot come to office due to transportation problem," "client cannot come to office during scheduled hours of agency or district," "client could not wait for service."

Finally, it was decided to differentiate between two kinds of referrals out: Type 1 (most appropriate service available elsewhere), and Type 2 (service requested is appropriate to agency, but not currently available). Type 2 was included as an early alert that the agency should consider services or programs not currently available, but which would be appropriate for the agency to deliver.

The second major decision had to do with information on financial disbursement. The executive staff of the agency wanted to know about the kinds of cases which received financial aid, the basis for its disbursement, and the specific type of aid given. These were accordingly included on the closing document. The amount of financial aid given was not made part of the system because the agency already had bookkeeping procedures which were tied in with the JFC accounting department.

The intake form is filled out by both the receptionist and the individual worker assigned the case. The worker fills out contact slip and closing form. Intake change is handled by worker where clinical information is concerned and by the clerical staff where administrative information is involved (such as transfer of a case to a new worker or district).

All documents are submitted for keypunching and computer input at the close of the month. During the following month errors are returned to workers and their corrections re-entered to the computer. Monthly reports are produced by the end of the month and forwarded to the appropriate recipients.

System Design

Non-technical persons involved in designing an information system typically tend to leave all technical consideration "to the expert." A rudimentary understanding of the computer side of an information system is well within the grasp of non-technical personnel.

Some knowledge of this area is particularly useful to the non-technical person in facilitating a better understanding of the capabilities, limitations, and procedures of computing. An overview of the technical structure of the SDIS is presented here in order to clarify those basic data processing considerations which form the framework of an information system. The discussion also stresses the relationship between agency policy and technical design.

Despite the complexity of detail involved in the data processing specification of an information system, there are really only four basic concepts involved: sort fields, master file, updating, and reporting.

Master File

The master file, like a paper file, consists of case records. The case record consists of case identifying information (ID and ID check) and a record of one or more "episodes." An epsode is an opening of a case. When the case closes this is a completed episode, otherwise it continues as an open episode. When the case reopens, a new episode begins. Thus, we are not limited to the most recent episode, but have the ability to analyze patterns of multiple openings and closings.

An episode contains all data from the intake form and the closing form (added when the case closes), as well as information developed from the contact slips. The contact slip contributes to the master file, the date of first contact, date of last contact, and cumulative counts of time spent and number of contacts for each type of contact listed on the contact slip.

Updating the Master File

Updating is the process by which the various forms add to or modify the information contained in the master file. For example, an intake form which indicates that the case is new would cause the creation of a new record, unless the system already has a case with the same case identifier, in which case an "error message" would be returned. On the other hand, if the case is said to be a reopened case, and there is no record of this identifier in the master file, another "error message" is returned. Similarly, a closing document cannot update an episode which is not yet open (or reopened).

The contact slips are used to update the cumulative count and time per modality as well as the dates of first and last contact of the current episode.

Reports

The master file is updated once a month when all documents filled out during the month are keypunched and input to the system. A program called "validate" locates errors (such as those mentioned above) and produces an error report. Once the errors are corrected (using a computer program called 'edit') the master file is then updated and the monthly reports are produced.

System Rules and Agency Policy

The errors programmed in the validation program were determined by the rules of the system. These rules were in turn based on the policies of the agency itself. A few such rules are discussed here for illustrative purposes:

(1) *An intake form must have at least one contact slip.* Casework activity must take place in order to open a case. Otherwise the intake becomes part of

the standard "no case made" file already maintained by the agency previous to starting the computerized system. From a systems point of view this saves the master file from being cluttered with non-cases by rejecting as errors those intakes not accompanied by contact slips.

(2) *Only one opening and one closing are allowed for a given case within the same month.* The original impetus for this rule came from the system designer in order to avoid an excessive data processing burden. It became clear in discussion with the agency personnel that this also made good casework sense. If a case opens, closes, and then reopens within the same month, it probably should not have been closed to begin with.

(3) *Contacts are recorded only for an open case.* This is a less obvious rule than is at first apparent. Workers will sometimes have a contact with a client after the case is closed. This rule reduces the temptation to continue contacts without reopening the case—a practice distinctly contrary to established agency policy.

At the end of the month all errors are sent back to the workers with messages such as "contact with unopened case," "intake of already open case," etc. When the errors have been corrected, the documents are re-submitted to the system so that the master file can be correctly updated.

Sort Fields and Reporting

All four documents begin with the same six pieces of information. These are called sort fields, and are used to organize the input data in such a way as to minimize processing costs. In addition, these sort fields make it possible to produce reports at various levels of specificity. The worker ID is used to produce a monthly summary of activity for each worker. In combination with the date of last contact and current date, the worker ID is used to produce a list of overdue cases (that is, cases which have had no activity for sixty days or more). The district sort field is used to sort the input data to produce district level caseflow reports and a summary of case activity for each district. The agency sort field separates the JFS data from the other agencies on the system (Jewish Big Brothers, Jewish Family Service of Santa Monica, and Jewish Vocational Service).

Buy or Build

Once the specifications for the system were agreed on, the task-group had to choose between purchasing an existing system or designing an original one. In order to reduce costs, a number of existing models were examined and ultimately rejected because they were not suitable. This includes the Statistical Package for the Social Sciences (SPSS) in Elliott R. Rubin, "The Implementation of an Effective Computer System," *Social Casework*, July, 1976, Vol.

57, No. 7, pp. 438–447. SPSS was found unusable because it is a "static" system. It sets up a complete "record," of data fed into it, but cannot easily alter this record once set up. For example, an agency using SPSS would have to cumulate activity over the life of the case (by hand) and then include the total as a part of the clinical record at the close of the case. We found this unacceptable because: (1) it involved unnecessary activity on the part of the worker in keeping track of case activity; (2) it would make monthly reports of caseflow and case activity impossible; and (3) it could not be used for other special applications. It is an excellent tool for the statistical analysis of data such as that exemplified by social surveys (precisely the purpose for which it is used in the Planning and Budgeting Department of the JF-C).

In the commercial field there are many applications which involve the creation and maintenance of a master file, procedures for updating it, and routines for producing required reports. Because none of these commercial systems were at all compatible with our needs, we found it necessary to create our own system. In sum, then, we decided not to compromise the requirements of our system in order to take advantage of an already existing package. Rather, we opted to develop a system that would meet the needs of the users.

Reports

The system produces two generic types of reports: standard monthly reports, and non-standard reports in response to specific requests. The monthly reports are run routinely and give an overview of the agency's activity for the month, while special reports are used to investigate a particular question in depth. In this section we will present some examples of each and will emphasize how they are related to the structure of the system itself. Because the applications of the system were a prime consideration in its design, an understanding of how reports are produced is useful to an agency contemplating the development of its own information system.

Routine Monthly Reports

At the end of the month the SDIS produces several standard reports which are described below.

General service report. This report gives a summary of caseflow by agency and district. Included are number of openings, closings, new cases, reopened cases, cases carried over from previous month, cases carried forward to next month, active cases, inactive cases, and overdue cases. "Overdue" cases are those which have been inactive for at least sixty days. This report provides the appropriate administrator(s) with an overview of the level of activity for the month.

Breakdown of active cases. This report, which is produced for both the agency and the districts, shows the number of cases which had 1 contact, 2–5 contacts, 6–10 contacts (etc.) during the month.

Breakdown by type of contact. This report presents the number of contacts and the total time spent on each type of contact during the month.

Breakdown of closed cases. This report presents the total number of contacts over the life of the case for cases which closed during the month. Because Jewish Family Service provides short term service, a majority of the cases should have had a cumulative total of five contacts or less.

Worker reports. Each worker receives three reports each month. A worker level version of the General Service Report is first, and shows individual caseflow. A worker level version of the breakdown of active cases report is second. This shows the time spent and number of contacts per type of contact for each worker. A detailed listing of the "overdue" clients in the individual worker's caseload is third. These worker level reports serve to give workers important feedback about their own activity during the month.

A Note on Confidentiality

Nowhere in the reports above or in any other part of the SDIS does the client's name ever appear. This is to ensure complete confidentiality. Only the client ID is listed on reports such as the overdue client report. In this respect the computerized system ensures greater confidentiality than the agency office where case files provide relatively open access.

Special Reports

The monthly case activity reports are produced dynamically—that is to say while updating the master file. Because input data is compared with the data in the master file, the monthly reports are produced as part of the master file update procedure. Special reports are static in the sense that they are based only on the contents of the master file. They are used to investigate various aspects of the client population, and in the next section we will present some examples of actual reports. Here we wish to describe how various pieces of information in the Master File can be used to create a special report.

The master file contains both the date of first contact and the date of last contact for the episode. Subtracting the former from the latter produces the duration of the case (measured in days). This would be done only for closed episodes, of course, as open episodes do not yet have the final date of contact. By bringing in date of birth we can compare case duration with age of client.

By subtracting the date of request for services from the date of first contact, we compute the waiting time from intake to initial casework activity. By cumulating time spent over the life of the episode, we can compute the cost of service.

We can compute the cost of service for age groups and for the various focus of service categories, or any other variable in the system. We could also compare the modalities most often used by the different age groups or focus of service categories. The inclusion of as simple an item as zip code makes it possible to carry out this sort of analysis on a geographic basis as well.

Clearly, all the possibilities are too numerous to describe here. In the initial design phase, careful consideration was given to the kinds of information to be used in special reports. The possibilities for in-depth analysis latent in the master file make the SDIS a valuable tool for evaluation and planning.

Sample Applications for Special Reports

Although the system is only nine months old at the time of this writing, it has already been used by both the Planning and Budgeting Department of Federation and the agency. Three such applications are discussed here: one requested by the Planning and Budgeting department, one requested by the agency, and one requested jointly.

The Planning and Budgeting department was interested in the volume and cost of service to the elderly (defined as 65 and older). Using date of birth to compute age, a report was prepared which provided the proportion of direct service time expended. Interestingly, in some districts the proportion of time taken up by the elderly was significantly greater than their proportion in the caseload, while in other districts the opposite was the case.

The program committee of JFS was charged with reviewing the district structure of the agency. One report run for this study compared the average time spent per case, the average duration of case (in days), and the average number of contacts per case in each district. Another report compared the focus of service and source of referral patterns for each district.

As the JFC of LA moves more toward decentralized planning and budgeting, both the agency and the Planning and Budgeting department will rely more heavily on a profile of the client population by area of the city. The availability of separate demographic data on the Jewish community of Los Angeles makes it possible to use the SDIS to compare the caseload of the agency with Jewish population of the city as a whole on the area by area basis.

Cost Effectiveness

The cost effectiveness of the SDIS can be evaluated four different ways. First, the absolute cost of the system comes to about $2.00/episode including worker time for filling out the forms. The average cost per episode in direct service comes to about $40/episode. The system cost is about five percent of direct service costs. A second approach is to compare the total cost of running the SDIS with the total agency budget. In this comparison the SDIS constitutes about one percent of the total budget, while informing the agency about too much of the remaining 99 percent is spent. A third approach is to compare the cost of the SDIS with the old manual system. To begin with, the old manual system could not handle the kinds of routine monthly reports produced by the SDIS, so comparison is better based on the special reports. Because of the time involved, the cost of producing just one special report could easily amount to a substantial proportion of the yearly cost of operating the system. Further, it is doubtful that such a report would be ready in time for it to be used, not to mention the increased accuracy of an automated system.

Finally, one should take into consideration the benefits of the system which cannot be given a cost figure. The ability of an agency to learn about itself is an intangible commodity, but the most significant benefit of the system.

Summary

In this paper we have briefly reviewed the process of developing an agency Service Delivery Information System in order to suggest a procedural model for other case work agencies considering such an undertaking.

We have tried to present not only an outline of steps, but the kinds of criteria used for making decisions about such a system. Particular attention was given to the technical structure of the system and the way in which technical considerations are included in developing a system.

An addition, reporting applications were selected which exemplify the utility of the system for the decision-makers who were involved in the design of the system. Attention was given to the production of reports from the information in the master file to evaluate the advantages of a flexible reporting capability and to suggest to the non-technical reader some of the ways in which the system combines data elements to produce required reports.

The small, medium sized, or even large agency may not have the funds available to produce such a system. However, a consortium of roughly similar agencies (from the point of view of structure and data processing) could divide the costs of developing a shared system, thereby reducing initial investment to a realistic amount. This in fact, is what we have accomplished by developing a shared system for the social casework agencies affiliated with the Jewish Federation council of Greater Los Angeles.

11. SYSTEMS DESIGN AND DOCUMENTATION: AN ESSENTIAL RELATIONSHIP FACILITATED VIA HIPO DIAGRAMS

Gunther R. Geiss, PhD

There are a number of essential considerations in the creation of any system regardless of which particular form the system takes, i.e., a human system, manual system, or an automated information system. These include: the acquisition of the hardware (furniture, office machines, computers, etc.); the acquisition of the software (policies, procedures, forms, programs, etc.); training staff; implementing and operating the system; and maintaining the system. Once the hardware acquisition decisions have been made, the principal focus shifts to the software and decisions regarding whether to design and develop new software, to modify existing software, to purchase ''off-the-shelf'' software and customize it, or to purchase custom made software. The major common thread here is documentation. Without complete documentation each of these activities and surrounding decisions becomes ill-informed and thus, presumably, poorly executed. In particular, evaluation and comparison of choices, training, and, especially, maintenance of the system are severely hampered by incomplete or non-existent documentation (Schoech & Schkade, 1980).

Despite its central place in the viability and effectiveness of the system, documentation often is given low priority under the pressure to complete a system design, during the stressful period of system implementation and conversion from previous procedures, and in the context of problem solving

Dr. Geiss is Associate Professor, School of Social Work, Adelphi University, Garden City, NY 11530.

and system modification. The consequences of this inattention to the importance of documentation are: an incomplete or non-existent record of the system—its purpose, concepts, design, methods and processes, and details; training achieved largely via informal methods of "hands-on" learning, and dependence upon oral sources of anecdotal material; maintenance which is extraordinarily expensive or ultimately impossible; and eventual abandonment of the system before its life cycle has been completed. This applies equally well to the agency's organization, structure, and policy, to service delivery programs, and computer based information systems.

Past Practices

The "flow diagram" of Goldstine and von Neumann (1963) was devised to aid the conceptualization and documentation of early computer programs. Its ubiquitous modern counterpart, the flowchart, is a set of standardized symbols interconnected to show either the flow of control, or the flow of data, in a particular system design, but not both. The flowchart tends to draw attention to the intricacies and details of problem solution to the detriment of the problem solution as a whole (Ledgard et al., 1979). Its general form tends to be narrow and long, and is thus best recorded on rolls of paper as opposed to the common sheet which requires many breaks in the chart. There is no particularly easy form of reference from sheet to sheet, or from module to submodule, or from chart to descriptive text. The general form of flowcharts, being largely at the discretion of the designer, does not demand, or even suggest, adherence to the principles of structured design (Ledgard et al., 1979), e.g., a single entry point and single exit for each system module. Lastly, flowcharts focus enough attention upon the details and intricacies that designs based upon flowcharts tend to develop from the bottom up, i.e., as a "Tinker-Toy" assemblage of simple units that then form the more complex units, or design by accretion of commonly available elements. Thus, flowcharts do not contribute as much to design and documentation as their frequent usage might imply; in fact, they impede good design and documentation.

Top-Down, Structured Design and HIPO Diagrams

Good systems design requires that primary focus remain with the problem, with the needs the systems must meet, and not with the details of how particular actions will be achieved. This orientation is referred to as top-down design (Yourdon, 1975). Simply put, top-down design takes the architect's view of a building—an arrangement of structure and space to meet a set of functional and aesthetic purposes. Its counterpart, bottom-up design, takes the bricklayer's view of the same building—as an assemblage of foundations, footings, bricks, stones and mortar which fulfill a given specification. To be sure that the stated problem is solved, and solved well, the focus must remain on the problem and its solution via the development of appropriate major units of process or procedure.

Structured design or structured programming (Dahl et al., 1973; Miller & Lindamood, 1973; Yourdon, 1975) combine the concept of top-down design with the construction of designs which are elaborations of the four fundamental elements: sequences of activities, repetitive operations or loops, decisions, and procedures (Grogono, 1980). Sequences are sets of activities which are performed in a particular order, e.g., intake, diagnosis and evaluation, and treatment. Loops are sets of activities which are performed repetitively until a particular end is achieved, e.g., repeatedly dialing a phone number until the desired party is reached. Decisions are those activities which are influenced by the data, e.g., client eligibility determination; and procedures are groups of activities that may be used frequently (modules or sub-routines), e.g., the intake procedure or the billing procedure. Structured design then imputes a higher value to the organization and clarity of a design than to efficiency of design or operation and "cute" solutions. The ultimate focus of structured design is on the readability (clarity) and maintainability (ease of revision) of the design.

It is important to note that designs in which the modules are essentially independent processes, i.e., they depend on each other only for inputs or outputs with no awareness of individual process steps within any module, permit independent and parallel module design. Thus, the "Chief Programmer" or "team programming" concepts become viable. That is to say, only the "Chief Programmer" or team leader need be concerned with module interrelationships; the teams or staff units need be concerned only with the development of the module to which they are assigned. The primary virtue of module independence is the facilitation of parallel rather than serial module development; and this reduces the overall development time via utilization of many teams, and it makes very large complex projects feasible. The secondary virtue is the facilitation of testing and operation of individual modules without the need for all modules to be operational.

Module independence is, of course, the goal to which many organizational arrangements strive—departmental or functional independence; and the assumption upon which many executives and staff operate.

A recent development that supports the utilization of top-down design and structured design is the Hierarchical-Input-Process-Output (HIPO) diagram (Katzan, 1976). The essence of the HIPO diagrams are two graphic or schematic elements: the hierarchical diagram (much like the common organization chart), and the input-process-output diagram. The hierarchical diagram, particularly, focuses attention on the problem via a top-down development of essentially independent modular units, while the input-process-output diagram draws primary attention to the inputs and outputs, and the process that links them.

Both diagrams illustrate the flow of both control and information. Finally, the method provides a numerical indexing scheme, ala the Dewey decimal cataloguing system, which links diagram to diagram, diagram to explanatory text, and module to submodule. Thus, it serves to reinforce good design practices, and to provide good documentation at the same time.

HIPO diagrams are not limited to the design and documentation of computer based systems, but they may be applied to the design of any system (administrative, service delivery, research, evaluation, etc.). The essential value of HIPO diagrams is in producing a design that solves the problem, a design which is understandable for ease in training, and a system which is maintainable for a longer service life.

An Illustration

The concepts of HIPO diagrams are best conveyed with an illustration. Consider the problem of tracking clients in an agency environment that includes both internal and purchased services, and of monitoring those services. The tracking system has as its objectives:

1. recording services needed by each client;
2. recording when, what, and by whom services are provided to the client;
3. recording the outcomes of service;
4. recognizing failures in service.

The services monitoring system has as its objectives:

1. recording individual and aggregate client data;
2. recording client service needs;
3. recording services provided;
4. reporting gaps in service;
5. reporting trends in clients, services and servers.

These systems should inform: individual case managers about the individual cases, and their caseload as a whole; supervisors about their case manager's caseload individually and collectively; and central administration about unit operations and aggregate operations. This information should be conveyed in separate but consistent report formats which are to be produced periodically, as well as upon demand. These reports should convey the status of individual cases, the status of particular caseloads, the status of reporting, trends in cases, caseloads, reporting and purchase of service utilization. Finally, it should be implementable over the range of options from a manual paper based system, through a batch processing computer system, and up to an interactive, distributed processing system.

Information from clients and servers (both internal and purchased) are to be gathered on precoded forms which include: a background report—brief description of client and presenting problems completed on first contact; an intake report—an elaborate report on the client, client's environment, and presenting problems; monthly service reports—reports by both internal and purchased service providers of services needed, services provided, services not available, case goals, and goal achievement; and an outcome report—a report filed on case termination which provides reasons for termination, goals and their level of achievement, assessment of present status of client, and a service summary.

The design and documentation of this system begins with the hierarchical diagram which describes the major functional units in the system. Figure 1 (HIPO 1.0) describes the Client Tracking and Services Monitoring System as a supervisory module or master program which offers a menu of functions— data entry, batch (periodic) report generation, and demand report generation. A unique rule of interpretation of the HIPO diagram is that entities at the same hierarchical level are read from left to right, and they will be executed in that logical sequence in actual operation. Thus, the choice of data entry from the master menu implies it will be followed subsequently by generation of batch reports, and then by generation of demand reports. The numerical indices in the lower right corner of each module also reflect this sequence of events.

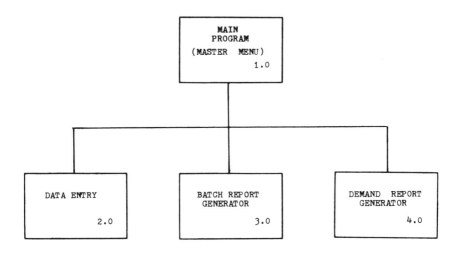

FIGURE 1 (HIPO 1.0)
CLIENT TRACKING AND SERVICES MONITORING SYSTEM

Figure 2 illustrates how a module (2.0 in this case) is elaborated by the subordinate HIPO diagram, and it shows how the numerical indices are assigned and how they reflect the subordination of modules to module 2.0. The relationship of modules may be determined by reading the figures or by examining their relative indices. Thus, unit 2.1.1 and unit 2.1.1.3 will be subunits of unit 2.1, and, in fact, unit 2.1.1.3 is a subunit of unit 2.1.1. For each module or unit to be elaborated there will be a HIPO diagram with the same index as the unit being elaborated. The focus on the problem and the top-down design process become quite evident.

The input-process-output diagram of Figure 3 is introduced when the design process reaches the stage where the elaboration of entities into operational steps is required. The diagram begins on the left with a listing of the inputs required for this process, the list of process steps follows in the center, and the resultant outputs on the right comprise this portion of the diagram.

The diagram is completed via the addition of the information flows (light arrows), and the control flows (dark arrows) as in Figure 4. The input consists of two distinct parts, the input reports, and the report log, these are processed through six steps to produce three output parts—the invalid reports, the sorted and logged reports, and the updated report log. Note that the sorted reports are returned to the process for entry into the report log. The heavy arrows show the flow of control from unit 2.1 to this unit (2.1.1) and then on to 2.1.2.

In summary, the hierarchical diagram identifies the relationship of modules via their hierarchical position as well as via their relative indices, and the flow of control is down to the left and then left to right at that level of the hierarchy. The input-process-output diagram lists the inputs, process steps, and outputs; and it indicates both the flow of control (heavy arrows) and the flow of information (light arrows). Outputs may be used as inputs to the same process that produced them, i.e., some outputs result from partial processing.

The remainder of this presentation will utilize the HIPO format.

Design Elaboration—2.0

Subunit 2.1 will control the report editing and coding process. This will be required to improve data quality in view of the tendency toward errors in interpretation and coding by those completing the forms. It also will serve to organize the reports for better throughput in subsequent processes.

Subunit 2.1.1 will initiate processing of reports by sorting them, validating basic identification data, logging valid reports, and rejecting invalid reports. The outputs are reports validated and sorted by type for subsequent processing, and invalid reports for return to the Case Manager.

Subunit 2.1.2 will review reports of one type at a time. The process is designed to verify responses against the codebook (instructions for form use with the allowable codes and interpretations), a consistency check (e.g.,

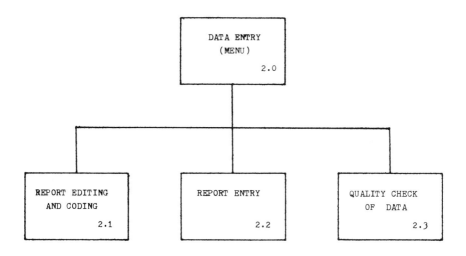

FIGURE 2 (HIPO 2.0)
DATA ENTRY SUBUNIT

responses for parents agree with reported number of parents in household), and a reasonableness check (e.g., childen's ages are commensurate with parent's ages). It will then complete coding entries (e.g., entry of proper codes in areas left blank by Case Manager) while verifying that entered codes are consistent with marked responses. Finally, any items which cannot be coded will be "red marked" with the reason they cannot be coded. This subunit will recycle until all reports have been processed.

Subunit 2.1.3. will review reports for responses to items which are written in or given as "other," and will produce a log of such responses for form redesign and/or user training. It will also correct the item coding in those cases where an existing code is applicable, or it will amend the codebook when a new code is introduced (e.g., a frequently occurring "other" response becomes an identifiable response). This subunit will be recycled until all reports have been reviewed.

Subunit 2.1.4 will review each report for acceptability on two criteria: (1) fatality level of the error; and (2) the count of non-fatal errors. It will also update the error file which may be used in management control and user training. This subunit will be recycled until all reports have been reviewed.

Given that these modules are essentially independent and that the inputs and outputs are clearly specified; then each module can be developed independently of the others, and will be functionally independent as well. That is, given the correct inputs it will produce the correct outputs regardless of how the inputs were created. Thus, modules can be tested independently by stimulating or furnishing the required inputs.

INPUT	PROCESS	OUTPUT
REPORTS: BACKGROUND INTAKE MONTHLY SERVICE (INTERNAL) MONTHLY SERVICE (PURCHASED) OUTCOME REPORT LOG CURRENT DATE	1. SORT REPORTS BY TYPE 2. SORT REPORTS BY SERVICE UNIT 3. SORT REPORTS BY WORKER 4. SORT REPORTS BY CASE NUMBER 5. VALIDATE CASE NUMBER VS. CASE NAME, WORKER I.D., SERVICE UNIT, PURCHASE OF SERVICE AGENCY, AND REPORT PERIOD 6. ENTER EACH REPORT INTO REPORT LOG WITH CURRENT DATE, AND DATE REPORT FILED	INVALID REPORTS RETURNED TO WORKER REPORTS SORTED FOR LOGGING AND EDITING UPDATED REPORT LOG

FIGURE 3 (HIPO 2.1.1)
AGGREGATION OF REPORTS BY TYPE

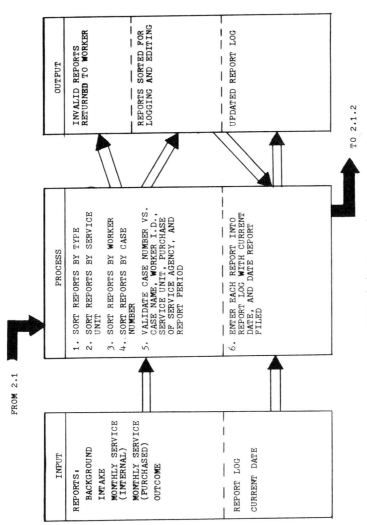

FIGURE 4 (HIPO 2.1.1)
AGGREGATION OF REPORTS BY TYPE

153

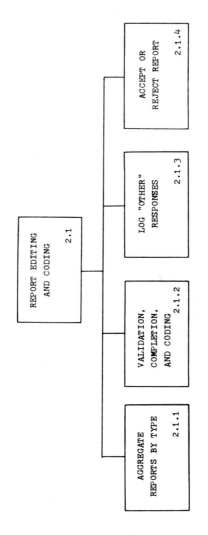

HIPO 2.1

In what follows, the HIPO diagrams will serve as the complete documentation, except where clarifying comments are very necessary. The pattern of interpretation should be well established by this point.

Design Elaboration—3.0

The Batch Report Generator will furnish the reports indicated in the HIPO diagrams. These reports will be formatted to provide exceptions first, and general data second. This will serve to draw attention to those areas most in need of correction and change. These exceptions should include:

—cases without contacts,
—cases without progress,
—services needed, but not provided,
—cases in which placements were made,
—placements which exceeded planned duration,
—placements completed before the planned date,
—cases with failed appointments,
—cases without POS service when agreed to,
—etc.

Reports will be consistent in format and content at the three organizational levels, for improved communication and staff involvement. The essential difference will be in coverage—all cases summarized for administration reports, only the Case Manager's cases summarized for the Case Manager, etc.

Process diagrams are not provided here because they will be implementation and machine dependent, i.e., they will depend upon decisions re: manual, batch, or interactive implementation: and the availablility of statistics packages, and data base management facilities.

Summary

Good system design and system documentation are intimately connected processes. Top-down and structured design processes are more likely to provide sound solutions to the initiating problem because of the focus on global issues as opposed to the minutiae of design. Both the documentation and these preferred design processes are facilitated via HIPO diagrams, while they tend to be impeded by the commonly used flowcharts.

HIPO diagrams consist of hierarchical figures which display the relationship of modules of activity; and input-process-output figures which display the inputs, process details, outputs, flow of information, and flow of control relative to one module. A numerical indexing system provides information regarding the hierarchical relationship of modules, and a link between the many figures and the descriptive text.

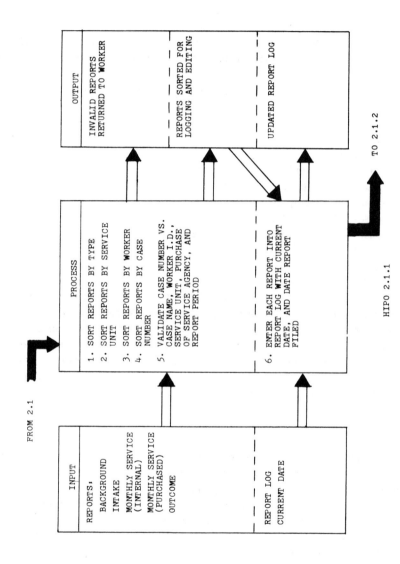

INPUT

REPORTS,

BACKGROUND

INTAKE

MONTHLY SERVICE
(INTERNAL)

MONTHLY SERVICE
(PURCHASED)

OUTCOME

REPORT LOG

CURRENT DATE

FROM 2.1

PROCESS

1. SORT REPORTS BY TYPE
2. SORT REPORTS BY SERVICE UNIT
3. SORT REPORTS BY WORKER
4. SORT REPORTS BY CASE NUMBER
5. VALIDATE CASE NUMBER VS. CASE NAME, WORKER I.D., SERVICE UNIT, PURCHASE OF SERVICE AGENCY, AND REPORT PERIOD
6. ENTER EACH REPORT INTO REPORT LOG WITH CURRENT DATE, AND DATE REPORT FILED

HIPO 2.1.1

OUTPUT

INVALID REPORTS
RETURNED TO WORKER

REPORTS SORTED FOR
LOGGING AND EDITING

UPDATED REPORT LOG

TO 2.1.2

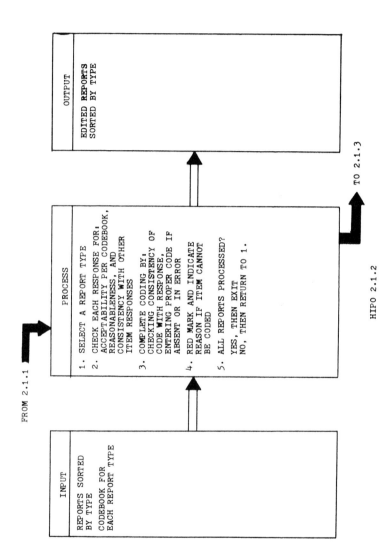

FROM 2.1.1

INPUT	PROCESS	OUTPUT
REPORTS SORTED BY TYPE CODEBOOK FOR EACH REPORT TYPE	1. SELECT A REPORT TYPE 2. CHECK EACH RESPONSE FOR: ACCEPTABILITY PER CODEBOOK, REASONABLENESS, AND CONSISTENCY WITH OTHER ITEM RESPONSES 3. COMPLETE CODING BY: CHECKING CONSISTENCY OF CODE WITH RESPONSE, ENTERING PROPER CODE IF ABSENT OR IN ERROR 4. RED MARK AND INDICATE REASON IF ITEM CANNOT BE CODED 5. ALL REPORTS PROCESSED? YES, THEN EXIT NO, THEN RETURN TO 1.	EDITED **REPORTS** SORTED BY TYPE

TO 2.1.3

HIPO 2.1.2

157

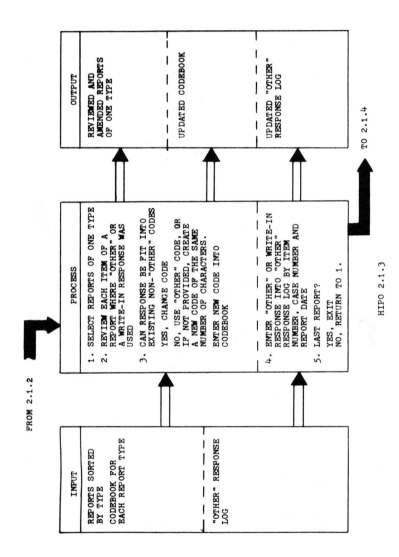

FROM 2.1.2

TO 2.1.4

HIPO 2.1.3

INPUT

REPORTS SORTED BY TYPE

CODEBOOK FOR EACH REPORT TYPE

"OTHER" RESPONSE LOG

PROCESS

1. SELECT REPORTS OF ONE TYPE

2. REVIEW EACH ITEM OF A REPORT WHERE "OTHER" OR A WRITE-IN RESPONSE WAS USED

3. CAN RESPONSE BE FIT INTO EXISTING NON-"OTHER" CODES

   YES, CHANGE CODE

   NO, USE "OTHER" CODE, OR IF NOT PROVIDED, CREATE A NEW CODE OF THE SAME NUMBER OF CHARACTERS.

   ENTER NEW CODE INTO CODEBOOK

4. ENTER "OTHER" OR WRITE-IN RESPONSE INTO "OTHER" RESPONSE LOG BY ITEM NUMBER, CASE NUMBER AND REPORT DATE

5. LAST REPORT?

   YES, EXIT
   NO, RETURN TO 1.

OUTPUT

REVIEWED AND AMENDED REPORTS OF ONE TYPE

UPDATED CODEBOOK

UPDATED "OTHER" RESPONSE LOG

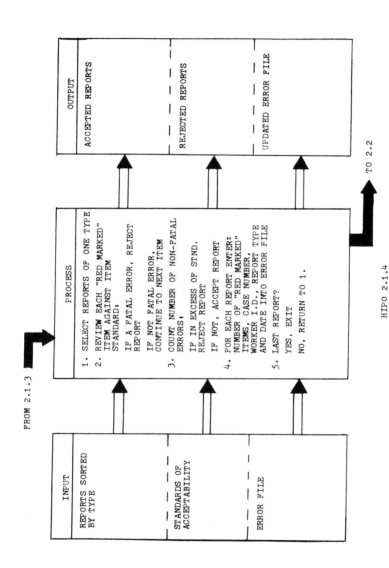

INPUT

REPORTS SORTED
BY TYPE

STANDARDS OF
ACCEPTABILITY

ERROR FILE

FROM 2.1.3

PROCESS

1. SELECT REPORTS OF ONE TYPE

2. REVIEW EACH "RED MARKED"
   ITEM AGAINST ITEM
   STANDARD:

   IF A FATAL ERROR, REJECT
   REPORT

   IF NOT FATAL ERROR,
   CONTINUE TO NEXT ITEM

3. COUNT NUMBER OF NON-FATAL
   ERRORS:

   IF IN EXCESS OF STND.
   REJECT REPORT

   IF NOT, ACCEPT REPORT

4. FOR EACH REPORT ENTER:
   NUMBER OF "RED MARKED"
   ITEMS, CASE NUMBER,
   WORKER I.D., REPORT TYPE
   AND DATE INTO ERROR FILE

5. LAST REPORT?

   YES, EXIT

   NO, RETURN TO 1.

TO 2.2

HIPO 2.1.4

OUTPUT

ACCEPTED REPORTS

REJECTED REPORTS

UPDATED ERROR FILE

159

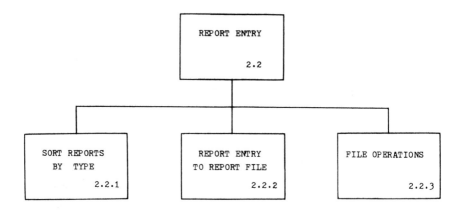

HIPO 2.2

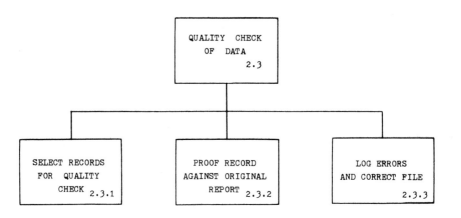

HIPO 2.3

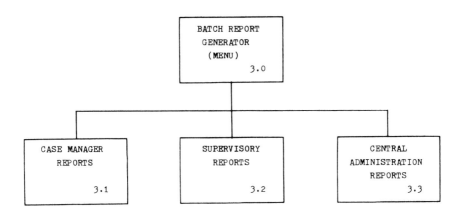

HIPO 3.0

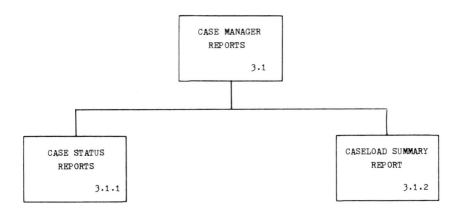

HIPO 3.1

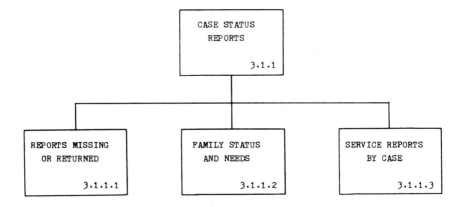

HIPO 3.1.1

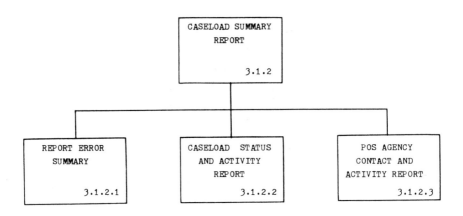

HIPO 3.1.2

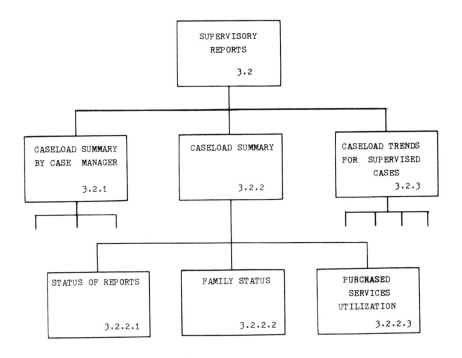

HIPO 3.2
(NOTE: REPORT STRUCTURE IS THE SAME FOR 3.2.1 & 3.2.2)

    While these techniques have developed within the context of computer programming and systems design, they are by no means limited to those activities. They can be applied to the design and documentation of a variety of systems in human services including the agency's organization and its service delivery processes.

    The application to the design of a client tracking and services monitoring system is explored in some detail with the HIPO diagram being the principle tool of documentation. Its utility becomes apparent when the amount of pure text required to achieve the same description is juxtaposed to the description given here. The descriptive effectiveness of the HIPO approach to design and documentation should contribute to improved training and improved system maintainability, while providing better problem solutions.

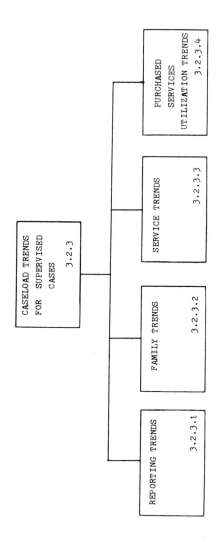

HIPO 3.2.3

CASELOAD TRENDS FOR SUPERVISED CASES
3.2.3

REPORTING TRENDS
3.2.3.1

FAMILY TRENDS
3.2.3.2

SERVICE TRENDS
3.2.3.3

PURCHASED SERVICES UTILIZATION TRENDS
3.2.3.4

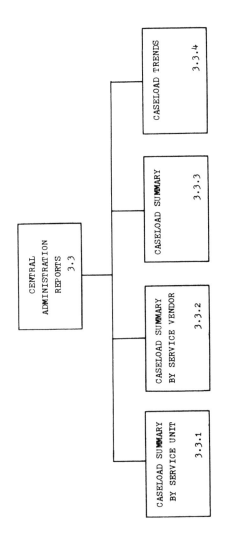

CENTRAL
ADMINISTRATION
REPORTS
3.3

CASELOAD SUMMARY
BY SERVICE UNIT
3.3.1

CASELOAD SUMMARY
BY SERVICE VENDOR
3.3.2

CASELOAD SUMMARY
3.3.3

CASELOAD TRENDS
3.3.4

HIPO 3.3

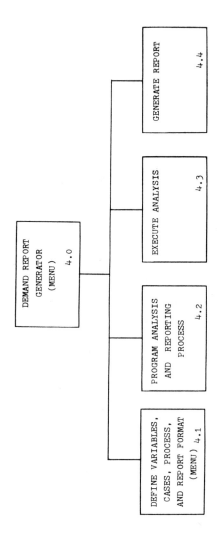

HIPO 4.0

REFERENCES

Dahl, O. J., Dykstra, E. W., & Hoare, C. A. R. *Structural programming*. New York: Academic Press, 1972.

Goldstine, H. H., & von Neumann, J. Planning and coding for an electronic computing instrument. *John von Neumann, Collected Works*, Vol. 5. New York: Pergammon Press, 1963.

Grogono, P. *Programming PASCAL*. Revised ed. Reading, MA: Addison-Wesley, 1980.

Katzan, H. Jr. *Systems design and documentation: An introduction to the HIPO method*. New York: Von Nostrand Reinhold Co., 1976.

Ledgard, H. F., Hveras, J. F., & Nagin, P. A. *PASCAL with style: Programming proverbs*. Rochelle Park, NJ: Hayden Book Co., 1979.

Miller, E. F. Jr., & Lindamood, G. E. Structured programming: Top-down approach. *Datamation*, 1973, *19*.

Schoech, D. J., & Schkade, L. L. What human services can learn from business about computerizaton. *Public Welfare*, 1980, *38*, 18–27.

Yourdon, E. *Techniques of program structure and design*. Englewood Cliffs, NJ: Prentice-Hall, 1975.

A NOTE FOR THE FIELD

COMPUTER USE IN SOCIAL SERVICES NETWORK

We are a group of human service professionals interested in computers and their use in services provision, research, and education. We are establishing a network whereby human service professionals with interests and needs in using computers can learn from each other by sharing ideas and concerns.

The network idea is simple. Members in the network send information to a central hub which puts it together in a newsletter and sends it back out. The network idea is realized as members read the newsletter, contact other members, and exhange information and ideas.

We have received support from the University of Texas at Arlington Graduate School of Social Work to send serveral issues of the newsletter free to anyone interested. Those who find the network useful and want to continue receiving the newsletter will be asked for a donation to cover the cost of printing and postage. We hope to send out 4 newsletters a year at approximately three month intervals.

If you are interested, send us information such as your name, occupation, mailing address, interests, current work with computers, skills, equipment you use, software you are familiar with, information needs, successes, mistakes, bibliographic materials, job available, relevant conferences, etc. Remember the old adage ''garbage in—garbage out'' holds especially true for a network. Please specify if you do not want information you provide used for other than network purposes (e.g., other organizations using the network mailing list).

Send your information to: Dick Schoech, School of Social Work, Uni-

169

versity of Texas at Arlington, Box 19129, Arlington, Texas 76019, and then tell your friends about the network.

Please join us.

Dick J. Schoech, PhD
School of Social Work
University of Texas at Arlington

Floyd Bolitho
Department of Social Work
Latrobe University, Bundoora, Victoria, Australia

H. John Staulcup
School of Social Work
University of Washington, Seattle

SELECTED BIBLIOGRAPHY RELATED TO THE USE OF COMPUTERS AND INFORMATION SYSTEMS IN THE ADMINISTRATION OF HUMAN SERVICES

Dick J. Schoech, PhD

Surveys, Review Articles, Bibliographies

Aldrich, R. F. *Health records and confidentiality: An annotated bibliography with abstracts.* Washington D.C.: National Commission on Confidentiality of Health Records, 1977.

Alexander, G. Terminal therapy. *Psychology Today*, 1978, *12*(4), 50–60.

Bellerby, L. J. *Patterns of information system growth in community mental health centers.* Unpublished doctoral dissertation, Portland State University, 1980.

Beschner, G. M., Sampson, N. H., & D'Amanda, C. D. (Eds.). *Management information systems in the drug field.* Washington, D.C.: DHHS, National Institute on Drug Abuse, Pub. No. (ADM) 79-836, 1979. (A collection of 7 articles, several on the state-of-the-art in drug abuse information systems.)

Boyd, L. H., Jr., Hylton, J. H., & Price, S. V. Computers in social work practice: A review. *Social Work*, 1978, *23*, 368–371.

Bowers, G. E., & Bowers, M. R. *Cultivating client information systems.* Washington, D.C.: DHHS, Office of Intergovernmental Systems, Project Share Human Service Monograph Series No. 5, June 1977.

Dr. Schoech is Assistant Professor, Graduate School of Social Work, University of Texas at Arlington, PO Box 19129, Arlington, TX 76019.

171

Hedlund, J. L., & Hickman, C. V. Computers in mental health: A national survey. *Journal of Mental Health Administration*, 1977, *6*(1), 30–52.

Hedlund, J. G., Vieweg, B. W., Cho, D. W., Evenson, R. C., Hickman, C. V., Holland, R. A., Vogt, S. A. Wolf, C. P., & Wood, J. B. *Mental health information systems: A state-of-the-arts report.* Columbia, MO: University of Missouri, Health Care Technology Center, October 1979.

Hedlund, J. L., Vieweg, B. W., Wood, J. B., et al. *Computers in mental health: A review and annotated bibliography.* Washington, D.C.: DHHS, NIMH, in press.

Johnson, J. H., Giannetti, R. A., & Nelson, N. M. The results of a survey on the use of technology in mental health centers. *Hospital and Community Psychiatry*, 1976, *27*, 387–391.

Johnson, J. H., Giannetti, R. A., & Williams, T. A. Computers in mental health care delivery: A review of the evolution toward interventionally relevant on-line processing. *Behavior Research Methods and Instrumentation*, 1976, *8*(2), 83–91.

Schnibbe, H. C., & Prascil, R. E. *State mental health statistical/management information systems.* Washington, D.C.: National Association of State Mental Health Program Directors, November 1978.

Schoech, D., & Arangio, T. Computers in the human services. *Social Work*, 1979, *24*(2), 96–102.

United Way of America. *Directory—data processing activity.* Report of the Data Processing Service Committee. Alexandria, VA: June 1977.

General References

Attkisson, C. C., Hargreaves, W. A., & Horowitz, M. J. (Eds.) *Evaluation of human service programs.* New York: Academic Press, 1978 127–215. (Three chapters on information systems.)

Bower, A. C., & Richardson, D. H. A computer-based data bank. *Mental Retardation*, *13*, 32–33.

Bowers, G. E., & Bowers, M. R. *The elusive unit of service.* Washington, D.C.: DHHS, Office of Intergovernmental Systems, Project Share Human Service Monograph Series No. 1, September 1976.

Brandon, D. H., & Segelstein, S. *Data processing contracts: Structure, contents and negotiation.* New York: Van Nostrand Reinhold Company, 1976.

Burch, J. G., Jr., Strater, F. R., & Grudnitski, G. *Information systems: Theory and practice* (2nd ed.). New York: John Wiley & Sons, 1979.

Carter, D. E., & Newman, F. L. *A client-oriented system of mental health service delivery and program management: A workbook and guide.* Washington, D.C.: U.S. Government Printing Office, DHHS Pub. No. (ADM) 76-307, NIMH Series C., No. 12, 1976.

Chelimsky, E. Welfare administration and the possibilities for automation. *Public Welfare*, 1973, *31*(3), 7–15.

Cohen, S. H., Noah, J. C., & Pauley, A. New ways of looking at management information systems in human service delivery. *Evaluation and Program Planning*, 1979, *2*, 49–58.

Crawford, J. L., Morgan, D. W., & Gianturco, D. T. (Eds.). *Progress in mental health information systems: Computer applications*. Cambridge: Ballinger Publishing Co., 1974.

Danzinger, J. N. The "skill bureaucracy" and intraorganizational control: The case of the data procesing unit. *Sociology of Work and Occupations*, 1979, *6*(2), 204–226.

Davidoff, I., Guttentag, M., & Offut, J. (Eds.) *Evaluating community mental health services: Principles and practices*. Washington, D.C.: DHHS Pub. No. (ADM) 77-465, NIMH, 1977, 81–173. (5 articles on management information systems.)

Donahue, J. H. Angell, E. Becher, A. L., Cingolani, J., Nelson, M., & Ross, G. E. The social service information system. *Child Welfare*, 1974, *53*(4), 243–255.

Eastwood, M. R., Meier, H. M. & Woogh, C. M. Information systems in psychiatry. *Psychological Medicine*, 1978, *8*, 181–184.

Ein-Dor, P., & Segev, E. *Managing management information systems*. Lexington, MA: D.C. Heath and Co., 1978.

Elias, M. J., Dalton, J. H., Cobb, C. W., Lavoie, L., & Zlotlow, S. F. The use of computerized management information in evaluation. *Administration in Mental Health*, 1979, *7*(2), 148–161.

Elpers, J. R., & Chapman, R. L. Management information for mental health services. *Administration in Mental Health*, 1973, 1, 12–25.

Fein, E. A data system for an agency. *Social Work*, 1975, *20*, 21–24.

Hargreaves, W. A., & Attkisson, C. C. (Eds.). *Resource materials for community mental health program evaluation* (2nd ed.). Washington, D.C.: DHHS Pub. No. (ADM) 75-230, NIMH, 1977. (9 articles on management information systems.)

Hirotaka, T., & Schmidt, A. H. New promise of computer graphics. *Harvard Business Review*, 1980, *58*(1), 122–131.

Hoshino, G., & McDonald, T. P. Agencies in the computer age. *Social Work*, 1975, *20*(1), 10–14.

Keen, P. G., & Morton, M. S. *Decision support systems: An organizational perspective*. Reading, MA: Addison-Wesley Publishing Co., 1978.

King, J. A. (Ed.) *The multi-state information system: Theoretical and practical issues*. Orangeburg, NY: Rockland Research Institute, 1979.

Klein, M. H., Greist, J. H., & Van Cura, L. J. Computers and psychiatry. *Archives of General Psychiatry*, 1975, *32*(7), 837–843.

Knesper, D. J., Quarton, G. C., Gorodezky, M. J., & Murray, C. W. A survey of the users of a working state mental health information system: Implications for the development of improved systems. In Orthner, F. H. (Ed.), *Proceedings: The second annual symposium on computer applications in medical care*. New York: Institute of Electrical and Electronics Engineers, 1978, 160–165.

Kraemer, K. L., Dutton, W. H., & Northrop, A. *The management of information systems*. New York: Columbia University Press, 1980.

Kraemer, K. L., & King, J. L. *Computers and local government: Vol. I - A manager's guide* and *Vol. II - A review of research*. New York: Praeger, 1977.

Levinson, S. E., & Liberman, M. Y. Speech recognition by computer. *Scientific American*, 1981, *244*(4), 64–76.

Lucas, H. C. Jr., *Information systems concepts for management*. New York: McGraw-Hill Book Co., 1978.

Nolan, R. L. Managing the crises in data processing. *Harvard Business Review*, 1979, *57*(2), 115–126.

————. On-line assessment and evaluation. *Behavior research methods and instrumentation*, 1977, *9*(2), 108–143. (A series of six articles on mental health information systems.)

Polivy, D., & Salvatore, T. Constraints on effective information system development and use in the voluntary human service sector. In the *Proceedings from the 14th Annual Conference of the Urban and Regional Information Systems Association*, Washington, D.C.: URISA, September, 1976, 57–68.

Roland, J. The microelectronic revolution. *The Futurist*, 1979, *13*(2), 81–90.

Schoech, D. J. *Computer use in human services: A guide to information management*. New York: Human Sciences Press, 1981.

Shelly, G. B., & Cashman, T. J. *Introduction to computers and data processing*. Fullerton, CA: Anaheim Publishing Co., 1980.

Sidowski, J. B., Johnson, J. H., & Williams, T. A. (Eds.). *Technology in mental health care delivery systems*. Norwood, NJ: Ablex Publishing, 1980.

Siegel, J. M. Automated management information systems. *Administration in Mental Health*, 1980, *8*(1), 46–55.

Slavin, S. (Ed.) *Social Administration*. New York: Haworth Press, 1978. (3 articles on information systems.)

Smith, T. S., & Sorensen, J. E. (Eds.) *Integrated management information systems for community mental health centers*. Washington, D.C.: DHHS Pub No. (ADM) 75-165, NIMH, 1974.

Uhlig, R. P., Farber, D. J., & Blair, J. H. *The office of the future: Communication and computers*. New York: North Holland, 1979.

Vail, H. The automated office. *The Futurist*, 1978, *12*(2), 73–78.

Volland, R. J., & German, P. S. Development of an information system: A means for improving social work practice in health care. *American Journal of Public Health*, 1979, *69*(4), 335–339.

Worthley, J. A. Computers and management: Taming the technological environment of public administration. *Public Administration Review*, 1978, *38*(3), 290–293.

Information System Design, Acquisition, Implementation, and Management

Bellerby, L., Dreyer, L., & Koroloff, N. *Information system improvements for mental health programs*. Portland, OR: Portland State University, Regional Research Institute for Human Services, MIS Curriculum Development Project, 1980. (A 3 volume workbook, Vol. I - Preparing for System Improvement, Vol. II - Planning Information System Improvements, and Vol. III - Managing the Design of System Improvements.)

Boyd, K. N., & Silver, E. S. *Factors affecting the development and implementation of information systems for social services*. Washington, D.C.: DHHS, Social and Rehabilitative Service, May 1975.

Chapman, R. L. *The design of management information systems for mental health organizations: A primer*. Washington, D.C.: U.S. Government Printing Office, DHHS Pub. No. (ADM) 76-333, NIMH Series C. No. 13, 1976.

Cobb. C. W. Problems and principles in the development of management information systems. *International Journal of Mental Health*, 1976–77, *5*(4), 103–120.

Cooper, M. *Guidelines for a minimum statistical and accounting system for community mental health centers*. Washington, D.C.: U.S. Government Printing Office, DHHS Pub. No. (ADM) 77-14, NIMH Series C. No. 7, 1977.

————. Documentation on the prototype community mental health center system design project. Springfield, VA: National Technical Information Service (NTIS), 1980. (Vol. 1., Feasibility of developing a prototype minicomputer CMHC management information system (PB 80-225915); Vol. 2., Summary of data elements and information necessary to satisfy CMHC program management reporting, and accountability requirements (PB 80-225907); Vol. 3., Requirements statement for the CMHC management information system (PB 80-224769); Vol. 4., Suggested system standard for the NIMH prototype management information system for CMHCs (PB 80-224-777); Vol. 5., Implementation guide for the NIMH prototype management information system for CMHCs (PB 80-224785); Vol. 6., System design for the NIMH prototype MIS for CMHCs: Processing logic (PB 80-224793); Vol. 7., System design for the NIMH prototype MIS for CMHCs: Data content and structure (PB 80-224801); Vol. 8., System design for the NIMH prototype MIS for CMHCs: Data content and structure appendix (PB 80-224819).

Dow, J. T. Designing computer software for information systems in psychiatry. *Computer and Biomedical Research*, 1975, *8*, 538–539.

Kupfer, D. J., Levine, B. G., & Nelson, J. A. *Mental health information system design and implementation*. New York: Marcel Decker, 1978.

Lowe, B. H., & Sugarman, B. Design considerations for community mental health management information systems. *Community Mental Health Journal*, 1978, *14*(3), 216–223.

Maypole, D. E. Developing a management information system in a rural community mental health center. *Administration in Mental Health*, 1978, *6*(1), 69–80.

Newman, F. L., & Sorensen, J. E. *The program director's guidebook for the design and management of client oriented systems*. Belmont, CA: Lifetime Learning, Wadsworth Publishers, Inc., 1981.

Paton, J. A., & D'huyvetter, P. K. *Automated management information systems for mental health agencies: A planning and acquisition guide*. Washington, D.C.: U.S. Government Printing Office, DHHS Pub. No. (ADM) 80-797, NIMH Series FN No. 1, 1980.

Percy, E. A. Incremental improvement of a community mental health center management information system. *Evaluation*, 1977, *4*, 205–207.

Rubin, E. R. The implementation of an effective computer system. *Social Casework*, 1976, *57*(7), 438–445.

Saver, A. R. *Procedures for operating a service delivery information system*. New York: Family Service Association of America, 1978.

Schoech, D. J., & Schkade, L. L. What human services can learn from business about computerization. *Public Welfare*, 1980, *38*(3), 18–27.

Squire, E. *Introducing systems design*. Reading, MA: Addison-Wesley, 1980.

St. Clair, C. H., Siegel, J. M., Caruso, R., & Spivack, G. Computerizing a community mental health center information system. *Administration in Mental Health*, 1976, *4*(1), 10–18.

Specific Applications

Cameron, J. C. Using a computer profile to assess quality of care in a psychiatric hospital. *Hospital and Community Psychiatry*, 1976, *27*(9), 623.

Davis, D., & Allen, R. The evolution of management information system in an outpatient mental health institute. *Administration in Mental Health*, 1979, *6*(3), 225–239.

Evenson, R. C., Sletten, I. W., Hedlund, J. L., & Faintich, D. M. CAPS: An automated evaluation system. *American Journal of Psychiatry*, 1974, *131*(5), 531–534.

Fanshel, D. Computerized information systems and foster care. *Children Today*, 1976, *5*(6), 14–18.

Gibelman, M., & Grant, S. The uses and misuses of central registries in child protective services. *Child Welfare*, 1978, *57*(7), 405–413.

Gifford, S., & Mayberry, D. An integrated system for computerized patient records. *Hospital and Community Psychiatry*, 1979, *30*, 532–535.

Gifford, S., Shaw, C., & Newkham, J. *Community health automated record and treatment system* (CHARTS). Unpublished manual, 1979. (Available from Heart of Texas Region Mental Health Mental Retardation Center, P.O. Box 1277, Waco, Texas 76703.)

Herson, J., et al. FP/MIS: A management information system for a community family planning clinic. *Medical Care*, 1977, *15*(5), 409–418.

Jaffee, E. D. Computers in child placement planning. *Social Work*, 1979, *24*(5), 380–385.

Johnson, J. H., & Williams, T. A. The use of on-line computer technology in a mental health admitting system. *American Psychologist*, 1975, *30*(3), 388–390.

Lehrer, B. E., & Daiker, J. F. Computer based information management for professionals serving handicapped learners. *Exceptional Children*, 1978, *44*, 578–585.

Luse, F. D. Use of computer simulation in social welfare management. *Administration in Social Work*, 1980, *4*(3), 13–22.

Maronde, R. F. Computer monitoring of psychotropic drug prescriptions. *Journal of Continuing Education in Psychiatry*, 1978, *39*, 11.

Meldman, M. J., Harris, D., Pellicore, R. J., & Johnson, E. L. A computer-assisted goal-oriented progress note system. *American Journal of Psychiatry*, 1977, *134*(1), 38–40.

Miller, G. H., & Willer, B. An information system for clinical recording, administrative decision making, evaluation and research. *Community Mental Health Journal*, 1977, *13*(2), 194–202.

Newman, F. L., Burwell, B. A., & Underhill, W. R. Program analysis using the client oriented cost outcome system. *Evaluation and Program Planning*. 1978, *1*, 19–30.

Paredes, A. Management of alcoholism programs through a computerized information system. *Alcoholism*, 1977, *1*(4), 304–309.

Poertner, J., & Rapp, C. A. Information system design in foster care. *Social Work*, 1980, *25*(2), 114–121.

Richey, B. The computer in a child care agency. *Child Welfare*, 1977, *56*(4), 259–270.

Schoech, D., & Schkade, L. L. Computers helping caseworkers: Decision support system. *Child Welfare*, 1980, *59*(9), 566–575.

Vondracek, F. W., Urban, H. B., & Parsonage, W. H. Feasibility of an automated intake procedure for human service workers. *Social Service Review*, 1974, *48*(2), 271–278.

Williams, T. A., Johnson, J. H., & Bliss, E. A computer assisted psychiatric unit. *American Journal of Psychiatry*, 1975, *132*, 1074–1076.

Wright, G. R. A system of service reporting: Its development and use. *Child Welfare*, 1972, *51*(3), 182–193.

Young, D. W. Computerized management information systems in child care: Techniques for comparison. *Child Welfare*, 1974, *53*(7), 453–463.

Zalkind, D., Zelon, H., Moore, M., & Kaluzny, A. Planning for management information systems in drug treatment organizations. *International Journal of Addictions*, 1979, *14*(2), 183–196.

Security, Privacy and Legal Considerations

Bank, R., & Laska, E. M. Protecting privacy and confidentiality in a multiple use, multiple user mental health information system. *Evaluation and Program Planning*, 1978, *1*(2), 151–158.

Collins, S. P. *Privacy: Concepts and issues*. Washington, D.C.: Library of Congress, Congressional Research Service, Issue Brief No. 1B74123, December 12, 1980.

Dial, O. E., & Goldberg, E. M. *Privacy, security, and computers—Guidelines for municipal and other public information systems*. New York: Praeger Publishers, 1975.

Gurthrie, D., Heighton, R., Keeran, C. V., & Payne, D. Data base and the privacy rights of the mentally retarded: Report of the AAMD task force on data base confidentiality. *Mental Retardation*, 1976, *14*, 3–7.

Harris, D. K., & Polli, G. J. Special report: Confidentiality of computerized patient information. *Computers and Medicine*, 1979. (Request report from American Medical Association, Department of Applied Medical Systems, 535 N. Dearborn, St., Chicago, IL 60610).

Laudon, K. C. Privacy and federal data banks. *Society*, 1980, *17*(2), 50–56.

Laska, E. M., & Bank, R. (Eds.) *Safeguarding psychiatric privacy: Computer systems and their uses*. New York: John Wiley & Sons, 1975.

Miller, A. R. The assault on privacy. *Psychiatric Opinion*, 1975, *12*(1), 6–14.

Noble, J. H. Protecting the public's privacy in computerized health and welfare information systems. *Social Work*, 1971, *16*(1), 35–41.

————. *Paperwork reduction act of 1980 (PL 96-511)*, December 11, 1980.

————. *Privacy act of 1974 (PL 93-579)*, December 31, 1974.

Rafferty, F., Beigler, J., et al. Model law on confidentiality of health and social service records. *American Journal of Psychiatry*, 1979, *136*(1), 138–148.

Reynolds, M. M. Threats to confidentiality. *Social Work*, March 1976, *21*(2), 108–113.

Wicklein, J. How Sweden keeps its computers honest. *The Progressive*, 1980, *44*(11), 34–38.

Wilson, S. J. *Confidentiality in social work: Issues and principles*. New York: The Free Press, 1978.

Information System Research, Evaluation, and Impacts

Adler, M., & DuFeu, D. Technical solutions to social problems: Some implications of a computer-based welfare benefits information system. *Journal of Social Policy*, 1977, *6*, 445–446.

Bauer, S. P. The impact of automation on public welfare systems. *Public Welfare*, 1973, *31*(1), 39–42.

Danzinger, J. N. Technology and productivity: A contingency analysis of computers in local governments. *Administration and Society*, 1979, *11*(2), 144–171.

Ein-Dor, P., & Segev, E. Organizational context and the success of management information systems. *Management Science*, 1978, *24*, 1064–1077.

Ein-Dor, P., & Segev, E. Strategic planning for management information systems. *Management Science*, 1978, *24*, 1631–1641.

Mason, R. O., & Mitroff, I. I. A program for research on management information systems. *Management Science*, 1973, *19*, 475–485.

Nolan, R. L., & Wetherbe, J. C. Toward a comprehensive framework for MIS research. *MIS Quarterly*, 1980, *4*(2), 1–19.

Norman, C. *Microelectronics at work: Productivity and jobs in the world economy.* Washington, D.C.: Worldwatch Institute (Paper 39), October 1980.

Offermann, L. R. Evaluating a computer-based information system in a CMHC. *Hospital and Community Psychiatry*, 1979, *30*(6), 379–383.

Quinn, R. E. The impact of a computerized information system on the integration and coordination of human services. *Public Administration Review*, 1976, *36*(2), 166–174.

Critical Perspective

Abels, P. Can computers do social work? *Social Work*, 1972, *17*(5), 5–11.

Agnew, N. M. Mental health systems: Tools, toys or weapons? *International Journal of Mental Health*, 1977, *5*(4), 32–38.

Danzinger, J. N. Computers, local governments, and the litany to EDP. *Public Administration Review*, 1977, *37*, 28–37.

Danzinger, J. N. The use of automated information in local government: A critical assessment. *American Behavioral Scientist*, 1979, *22*(3), 363–392.

Dutton, W. H., & Kraemer, K. L. Automating bias. *Society*, 1980, *17*(2), 36–42.

Dutton, W. H., & Kraemer, K. L. Technology and urban management: The power payoffs of computing. *Administration and Society*, 1977, *9*(3), 305–340.

Herzlinger, R. Why data systems in nonprofit organizations fail. *Harvard Business Review*, 1977, *55*(1), 81–86.

Kelley, V. R., & Weston, H. B. Computers, costs, and civil liberties. *Social Work*, 1975, *20*(1), 15–19.

Kraemer, K. L. Local government, information systems, and technology transfer: Evaluating some common assertions about computer applications transfer. *Public Administration Review*, 1977, *37*, 368–382.

Kraemer, K. L., & Dutton, W. H. The interests served by technological reform: The case of computing. *Administration and Society*, 1979, *11*(1), 80–106.

Kraemer, K. L., & King, J. L. *Computers, power and urban management: What every local executive should know*. Beverly Hills: Sage Publications, Inc., 1976.

Noah, J. C. Information systems in human services: Misconceptions, deceptions, and ethics. *Administration in Mental Health*, 1978, *5*(2), 99–111.

Sullivan, R. J. Human issues in computerized social services. *Child Welfare*, 1980, *59*(7), 401–406.

Weizenbaum, J. *Computer power and human reason*. San Francisco: W. H. Freeman and Co., 1976.

Woodridge, S., & London, K. *The computer survival handbook* (Rev. ed.). Ipswich, MA: Gambit, 1980.

Small Systems

Abernathy, W. B. The microcomputer as a community mental health public information tool. *Community Mental Health Journal*, 1979, *15*(3), 192–202.

Osborne, A., & Cook, S. *Business system buyer's guide*. Berkeley, CA: Osborne/McGraw Hill, 1981.

Schoech, D. A microcomputer based human service information system. *Administration in Social Work*, 1979, *3*(4), 423–440.

Shaw, D. R. *Your small business computer*. New York: Van Nostrand Reinhold Co., 1981.

Sipple, C. J., & Dahl, F. *Computer power for the small business*. Englewood Cliffs, NJ: Prentice-Hall, 1979.

Taylor, J. B., & Gibbons, J. *Microcomputer applications in human service agencies*. Washington, D.C.: DHHS, Office of Intergovernmental Systems, Project Share Human Services Monograph Series No. 16, November 1980. (Also available as a Sage Human Service Guide, Beverly Hills: Sage Publications, 1980.)

Whinston, A. B., & Holsapple, C. W. DBMS for micros. *Datamation*, 1981, *27*(4), 165–167.

The "Systems" Context of Information Systems

Gall, J. *Systemantics: How systems work and especially how they fail.* New York: Pocket Book, 1975.

Gruber, M. (Ed.) *Management systems in the human services.* Philadelphia: Temple University Press, 1981. (4 articles on management information systems.)

Schoderbek, Schoderbek, & Kefalas. *Management systems: Conceptual considerations* (Rev. ed.). Dallas: Business Publications, 1980.

Van Gigch, J. P. *Applied general systems theory* (2nd ed.). New York: Harper & Row, 1978.

Education and Curriculum

Anderson, C. M. Information systems for social welfare: Educational imperatives. *Journal of Education for Social Work*, 1975, *11*(3), 16–21.

Athey, T. A. Computer information systems curriculum development *Interface/The Computer Education Quarterly*, 1981, *2*(4), 20–24.

Davis, G. B. Forthcoming update of the ACM information system curriculum. *Interface/The Computer Education Quarterly*, 1981, *3*(1), 15–17. (Two efforts are occuring to develop a model curriculum for programs in information systems. The Davis article discusses one, the Athey article discusses the other.)

Flynn, M. L. Computer-based instruction in social policy: A one-year trial. *Journal of Education for Social Work*, 1977, *13*, 52–59.

Goldstein, H. K., & Dedmon, R. A computer-assisted analysis of input, process and output of a social work education program. *Journal of Education for Social Work*, 1976, *12*(2), 17–20.

Reeves, G. R., & Bussom, R. S. Information systems curriculum. *Journal of Systems Management*, 1979, *30*(3), 18–21.

Schwartz, M. D. A device integrating computer assisted and videotape instruction. *Computers in Psychiatry/Psychology*, 1978, *1*(3), 10. (A bi-monthly newsletter available from 26 Trumbull St., New Haven, CT.)

INDEX

In addition to subjects covered in *Applying Computers in Social Service & Mental Health Agencies: A Guide to Selecting Equipment, Procedures and Strategies*, this index incorporates items published in issues 1 and 2 of *Administration in Social Work*, volume 5.

Book Reviews